WHAT ARE YOU
HUNGRY FOR?

*The Essential Spontaneous Fulfillment of Desire: The Essence of Harnessing
the Infinite Power of Coincidence*

The Future of God

The Lords of Light

The Love Poems of Rumi
(edited by Deepak Chopra; translated by Deepak Chopra and Fereydoun Kia)

The Seven Spiritual Laws of Success: Pocketbook Guide to Fulfilling Your Dreams

The Seven Spiritual Laws for Parents

The Seven Spiritual Laws of Superheroes (with coauthor Gotham Chopra)

The Seven Spiritual Laws of Yoga (with coauthor David Simon)

The Soul in Love

The Soul of Leadership

The Spontaneous Fulfillment of Desire

The Ultimate Happiness Prescription

Unconditional Life

Walking Wisdom: Three Generations, Two Dogs, and the Search for a Happy Life
(contributor; authored by Gotham Chopra)

Why Is God Laughing?

FOR CHILDREN

On My Way to a Happy Life
(with coauthor Kristina Tracy, illustrated by Rosemary Woods)

You with the Stars in Your Eyes (illustrated by Dave Zaboski)

FROM DEEPAK CHOPRA BOOKS

Infinite Potential by Lothar Schäfer

Science Set Free by Rupert Sheldrake

Supernormal: Science, Yoga, and the Evidence for Extraordinary Psychic Abilities
by Dean Radin

The Generosity Network by Jennifer McCrea and Jeffrey C. Walker

DEEPAK CHOPRA

WHAT ARE YOU HUNGRY FOR?

The Chopra Solution to
Permanent Weight Loss,
Well-Being, and
Lightness of Soul

HARMONY

BOOKS · NEW YORK

Library of Congress Cataloging-in-Publication Data is available upon request.

ISBN 978-0-7704-3723-7
eBook ISBN 978-0-7704-3722-0

Printed in the United States of America

Book design by Chris Welch
Cover photography by David Malan/Getty Images

1 3 5 7 9 10 8 6 4 2

First Paperback Edition

Contents

PART TWO
RAISING YOUR CONSCIOUSNESS

PART THREE
RECIPES FROM THE CHOPRA CENTER KITCHEN

OVERVIEW:

AWARENESS AND WEIGHT LOSS

Why This Will Work
for You

At this moment there's a groundswell that is changing people's lives. It can be sensed from the headlines. A former president, shocked by suffering an early heart attack, announces that he has become a vegan. That's an amazing statement, and to back up his conversion, Bill Clinton tells everyone how good he feels—and looks. On another front, an extensive study in Spain finds that people who eat a Mediterranean diet high in fish, nuts, and olive oil can reduce the incidence of heart attacks by one-third. This is the biggest dietary finding in years. Everyone who was weaning themselves off red meat is medically vindicated.

The groundswell is moving on many other fronts. The toxins present in processed and manufactured food are less and less acceptable. *Organic* has become a mainstream word. More people than ever are becoming vegetarians, a lifestyle whose benefits have been known for a long time. (In one poll, half of British women described themselves as basically vegetarian.) In a sustainable world, there's no room for the polluting effect of pesticides and herbicides. People are waking up to a new reality, and a completely new way of eating has quickly emerged.

I got swept up in the groundswell about five years ago. I was already a "good" eater. My diet didn't include much red meat, and

I had long ago curbed obvious toxins like alcohol and tobacco. I enjoyed what I ate, and I ate what I enjoyed. But as I looked around at the medical literature, new findings were emerging every day. All kinds of links were being made between sugar and obesity, alcohol and disturbed sleep rhythms, simple carbohydrates and diabetes— and many of these findings affected being overweight.

Evidence was piling up that pointed in only one direction. I needed to find the ideal diet, because there was every good reason to. Only habit and neglect were keeping me from maximizing the connection between food, body, and mind.

Not to mention that I was carrying 20 extra pounds.

Despite my "good" eating, I had become a statistic, joining the two-thirds of Americans who are either overweight or obese. I became a statistic despite the fact that I had medical training, motivation, reasonably good habits, no major toxins, and access to any food I wanted. I also knew that going on a diet was futile—look at the numerous studies that prove, over and over, that the rebound effect makes you regain the weight you lost on your diet, and then 5 or 10 pounds more. The surplus pounds are your body's way of saying, "You tried to deprive me. Don't do it again."

My solution was to adopt the ideal diet, and I did it more or less overnight. There was no reason not to, given all the medical evidence I knew.

I eliminated all processed foods.

I ate the purest foods, always natural, as much organic as possible.

Already a nondrinker, I also eliminated fermented foods like cheese.

I gave up refined white sugar.

I drastically cut back on salt.

I gave up red meat, mostly eating chicken and fish but moving in the direction of being a vegetarian.

I drank pure water.

I paid attention to getting proper sleep.

Because everything is connected, something like getting a good night's sleep was part of my new way of eating. Lack of sleep throws off the balance between two hormones (leptin and ghrelin) responsible for making you feel hungry and full. People who don't sleep well overeat easily when their body stops sending the right hormonal messages. Belly fat disturbs the same hormones. And what you end up with is a self-perpetuating cycle that is not only unhealthy but potentially dangerous.

I didn't worry that I was becoming a purity fanatic. Nothing in my new eating was imposed. I wasn't motivated by worry or fear. The simple fact is that "normal" eating, American style, has gone to unhealthy extremes. The average American consumes 150 pounds of sugar a year, a grotesque amount of empty calories that wreak havoc on insulin levels and blood sugar. As for our addiction to processed foods, which account for 70 percent of what Americans eat, take a look at your local supermarket. There are whole aisles devoted to cookies, crackers, other snack foods, soda pop, frozen pizza, and ice cream. Economics rule, and if those foods didn't sell in abundance, they wouldn't get all that shelf space.

What's *not* extreme is to eat naturally, based on the best medical knowledge available. That's what the groundswell has been all about. Attention must be paid, and for the longest time our society hasn't been paying attention to the distorted way we eat.

I was pursuing "awareness eating." All the steps I took made me feel very good. My body felt lighter, even before I dropped 19 pounds, which came off effortlessly. I stopped doing unconscious things like taking cell phone calls during a meal—why not fully enjoy what you're eating? I didn't deprive myself either. Every meal was satisfying because my eating was now in tune with my body, and this in turn raised my mood level. Although I've always been an energetic person, I had energy and buoyancy as never before.

But the most gratifying thing was other people's response. When I talked about awareness eating, they nodded. Most had already been going along the same path that I was on. The groundswell was real and growing. Standing back, I saw that a tipping point had been reached. Collective consciousness had gotten the message.

When I sat down to write this book, I had confidence that many more people want to walk this new path. They didn't need to be coaxed into new beliefs, because healthy eating is already their goal. Yet certain things hold them back.

Bad habits and old conditioning.
Fear of change and family pressure not to change.
A stubborn belief that the next diet will work.
Discouragement about being overweight.
A history of not losing weight.
Hunger cravings, especially for salty, sweet, and fatty foods.
Time pressure, which makes it easy to reach for processed foods and snacks, and to make a quick stop at McDonald's.

It's a formidable list. These are huge obstacles in the lives of millions of people. In fact, it's amazing that a new way of eating has managed to become so popular—just look at television advertising, which uses buzzwords like *natural*, *light*, and *nutritious* to sell almost nothing but processed food, while the advertising for fresh fruits and vegetables, whole grains, and organic produce is next to nil.

To get past the obstacles that have led to your weight gain, whether it's a little or a lot, I'm not going to repeat the same advice about healthy eating that has existed for decades. The advice is all good. What's missing is how to change. Awareness is the key, because we have all been trained through massive conditioning to damage our bodies in the following ways:

Eating unconsciously, not caring what's in our food.

Losing control over our appetite.

Opting for bigger and bigger portions.

Using food for emotional reasons, e.g., to soften the stress of daily life.

Reaching for the fastest food that will satisfy our cravings.

All of these obstacles begin in one place: the mind. The body is a physical reflection of the choices you make over a lifetime. Knowledge is important, but adding more good advice isn't the solution to healthy eating. The solution is to transform your awareness.

I decided to show people how transformative awareness works, how they can achieve it, and why. Otherwise, the best advice, even when it leads to improved eating, will still leave us enclosed in limited notions of our bodies. Being a rigidly "good" eater who follows a set of rules and never deviates isn't a happy situation, either. But with transformed awareness, all of your ingrained, self-destructive behaviors can be changed easily. You can't control what you aren't aware of. If you had a rock in your shoe, you'd remove it immediately. The signals of pain tell you instantly that something is wrong. Eating poorly isn't like that. More often than not, it sends no pain signals, and the harmful effects often happen invisibly, gradually, and out of sight. You must gain a new level of awareness in order to notice what's going wrong inside you. Only then can you proceed to change it.

So, if you're overweight or feeling sluggish, or if your energy levels are low or you are unhappy about your body image, remembering how much better you looked and felt when you were younger, this book is for you. It will bring many surprises and discoveries—chief among them is that ideal weight is the most natural state you can be in. Your body can become your ally in finding a better way to live, reaching beyond weight loss. Awareness reveals many unexpected solutions, what I call applied wisdom.

Let's get down to it—the journey is exciting, and you can join the groundswell with real enthusiasm, knowing how much better you will look and feel.

Eating, Weight, and Hunger

If you want to return to your ideal weight, two choices face you. You can go on a diet or do something else. This book is about that something else. Dieting involves the wrong kind of motivation, which is why it rarely leads to the desired goal. You are taking the route of self-denial and doing without. Every day on a diet involves struggling against your hunger and fighting for self-control. Is there a more unsatisfying way to live?

Weight loss needs to be satisfying in order to succeed—this is the "something else" that works after dieting has failed. If you bring the body's hunger signals back into balance, your impulse to eat becomes your ally instead of your enemy. If you trust your body to know what you need, it will take care of you instead of fighting back. It's all about getting the messages straight that connect mind and body.

Medically, I was trained to analyze hunger in terms of the rise and fall of certain hormones. Hunger is one of the most powerful chemical messages sent by the body to the brain. It shouldn't happen that a person can feel hungry right after eating a meal or that having a snack in the afternoon should lead to a second snack or a third. But I've experienced these things—as have millions of people—which means that the *experience of hunger* can exist even when the need for food doesn't.

It's this experience of hunger that you need to change when you find yourself overeating. Cravings and false hunger aren't the same as giving your body the fuel it needs. Your body isn't like a gas-guzzling car. It's the physical expression of thousands of messages that are being sent to and from the brain. In the act of eating, your self-image is involved, along with your habits, conditioning, and memories. The mind is the key to losing weight, and when the mind is satisfied, the body quits craving too much food.

A mind-body approach will work for you because it asks you for only one thing: *Find your fulfillment.* To be fulfilled is something that food alone can't do. You must nourish:

- the body with healthy food
- the heart with joy, compassion, and love
- the mind with knowledge
- the spirit with equanimity and self-awareness

With awareness, all of these things become possible. But if you neglect them, they move further and further out of reach.

It sounds like a paradox, but to lose weight, you need to fill yourself. If you fill yourself with other kinds of satisfaction, food will no longer be a problem. It was never meant to be. Eating is a natural way to feel happy. Overeating isn't. For centuries life has been celebrated at feasts, and some of these celebrations, such as wedding banquets and retirement dinners, can be the highlight of a person's life. What child doesn't brighten up when the birthday cake appears? But the delight that food brings makes overeating a peculiar and unique problem. Feeling happy, which is good for you, morphs into something that's bad for you.

At this moment you fall somewhere on the sliding scale that connects food with happiness:

Normal eating $\longrightarrow$ *Overeating* $\longrightarrow$ *Cravings* $\longrightarrow$ *Food Addiction*

Eating normally feels good.

Overeating feels good in the moment but leads to bad results in the long run.

Giving in to cravings doesn't feel good at all—remorse, guilt, and frustration set in almost immediately.

Being addicted to food brings suffering, declining health, and total lack of self-esteem.

The slippery slope to becoming overweight starts with something that's actually positive: the natural goodness of food. (You can't say the same about drugs and alcohol, which can be toxic substances even when a person isn't addicted to them.) Food nourishes us, and when eating goes wrong, we are torn between short-term pleasure (such as a delicious bite of chocolate ice cream) and long-term pain (the many drawbacks of being overweight for years at a time).

So why does normal eating start to slide into overeating? The simple answer: lack of fulfillment. You start overeating to make up for a lack somewhere else. Looking back on my medical residency, when I was still in my twenties, I can see now how bad eating habits insinuate themselves. I'd come home from a grueling shift at the hospital feeling stressed out. My mind was still filled with a dozen cases. Some patients were still in jeopardy. What awaited me at home was a loving wife and a home-cooked meal.

In terms of getting enough calories, sitting down to dinner met all the requirements. You had to look at the human situation to see the hidden problems. I had hit the coffee machine and grabbed snacks on the run at work. From lack of sleep I didn't really notice what I was eating. The minute I walked in the door I usually had a drink, and there was a half-empty pack of cigarettes lying around somewhere.

In the seventies I was a normal working male following the same habits as every other young doctor I knew. I counted myself extremely fortunate to have such a loving wife and two beautiful babies at home. But the ravenous way I dug into a nourishing home-cooked dinner, combined with all the other signs of stressed eating, was setting a pattern that was desperately wrong. Ironically, even back then I considered myself pretty aware.

What turned the corner was becoming much more aware—the solution I'm proposing in this book. No matter how much it gets abused, the body can restore balance. The first rule is to stop interfering with nature. In its natural state, the brain controls hunger automatically. When your blood sugar falls below a certain level, messages are sent to an almond-sized region of the brain known as the hypothalamus, which is responsible for regulating hunger. When it receives messages of decreased blood sugar, your hypothalamus secretes hormones to make you feel hungry, and when you've eaten enough, the hormones reverse, making you no longer hungry. This feedback loop between blood and brain operates on its own, as it has for millions of years. Any animal with a spinal cord (vertebrate) has a hypothalamus, which makes sense, because hunger is so basic.

But in humans, hunger can get interfered with quite easily. The way we feel emotionally can make us ravenous or unable to eat at all. We can be distracted and forget to eat, or we can be obsessed and think about food all day. However, we are always in search of satisfaction. There are lots of things you can fill up on besides food. Desire comes from needs, starting with the most basic ones:

Everyone needs to feel safe and secure.
Everyone needs to feel nurtured.
Everyone needs to feel loved and appreciated.
Everyone needs to feel that their life is relevant and meaningful.

If you have filled these needs, food will be just one delight out of many. But countless people turn to overeating to substitute for what they really want. It becomes a game of switch-up, and often they don't even see what's happening. Is that the situation you find yourself in? Here are some common indicators.

You don't feel secure unless you are dulled by eating too much. Dullness brings a kind of calm that lasts a short while.

You don't feel nurtured except when your taste buds are over-stimulated with sugar, salt, and fat.

You don't feel loved and appreciated, so you turn eating into "giving myself some love."

Your life lacks meaning, but at least when you eat, the emptiness inside can be ignored for a little while.

If you stop focusing so hard on diet and calories, you can see that the story of overweight in America is the story of missed fulfillment. We have the best foods in the world at our disposal, but we gorge on the worst. We have blessed opportunities to grow and evolve, but instead we feel empty.

My goal is to bring you to a state of fulfillment. Once that begins to happen, you will stop eating for the wrong reasons. The solution is simple but profound: To lose weight, every step of the way must be satisfying. You don't have to psychoanalyze yourself; you can stop obsessing about your body and dwelling in disappointment and frustration. There is only one principle that applies: *Life is about fulfillment.* If your life isn't fulfilled, your stomach can never supply what's missing.

"What Am I Hungry For?"

Everyone's life story is complicated, and the best intentions go astray because people find it hard to change. Bad habits, like bad memories, stick around stubbornly when we wish they'd go away. But you have a great motivation working for you, which is your desire for happiness. I define happiness as the state of fulfillment, and everyone wants to be fulfilled. If you keep your eye on this, your most basic motivation, then the choices you make come down to a single question: "What am I hungry for?" Your true desire will lead you in the right direction. False desires lead in the wrong direction. You can take a simple test to prove this to yourself: The next time you go to the refrigerator for something to eat, stop for a second. What's making you reach for food? There are only two answers:

1. You're hungry and need to eat.
2. You're trying to fill a hole, and food has become the quickest way to do that.

Modern medicine has quite a lot of knowledge about the "triggers" that set off the impulse to eat. Your body secretes hormones and enzymes connecting the hunger center in your brain with the stomach and digestive tract. When you were a baby, this was the only kind of trigger you responded to. You cried because you were hungry. Now the reverse might be true: When you feel like crying, you get hungry.

Over a lifetime, we create new triggers that a baby could never anticipate. Depression is a well-known trigger for overeating. So are stress, sudden loss, grief, repressed anger—and there are many others. Which ones are you most vulnerable to? You probably have only a vague idea. Most people are unaware when their eating behavior is being triggered, because triggers are often unconscious—that's what makes them so powerful. You respond automatically without thinking.

Quiz:
What Triggers You to Overeat?

The most common triggers for overeating appear in the following checklists. Some are easier to overcome than others. Look at the lists and check the most common causes that make you eat *even when you're not hungry*. Mark as many items as you feel apply to you.

Group A: *I tend to overeat if*
___ I'm busy or distracted at work.
___ I'm rushed and on the go.
___ I'm tired. I haven't had enough sleep.
___ I'm with other people who are eating.
___ I'm out at a restaurant.
___ I'm in front of the TV or computer and need something to do with my hands.
___ I have a plate of food in front of me, and I feel I must clean my plate.

Group B: *I tend to overeat if*
___ I'm depressed.
___ I'm lonely.
___ I'm feeling unattractive.
___ I'm feeling anxious or worried.
___ I'm having negative thoughts about my body.
___ I'm under stress.
___ I want to be comforted.

Rating Yourself
If all or most of the items you checked come from Group A, your triggers are the easiest to overcome. You need to pay more attention to your eating habits, but that should be relatively easy. You can catch

yourself eating when you're not hungry because your main problem is distraction. Once you focus on one thing at a time—the meal in front of you—you will bring inattentive eating under control.

If all or most of the items you checked come from Group B, you are hungry for something else besides food, and paying attention to those things will be your best way to lose weight. One important thing is not going on a diet. Your pathway isn't deprivation; it's to find satisfaction in things other than eating.

Action Step:
Notice Your Trigger Before You Eat.

Now that you know your triggers, you can monitor them. You don't have to fight against your hunger, just give your brain enough time to make a choice. Instead of robotically reaching for food, which is a reaction that comes automatically, let yourself find a way to choose what you really want. At first, this involves a simple moment of mindfulness, or self-awareness, as follows:

Any time you are about to eat outside mealtime, go through the following simple steps:

1. Pause and take a deep breath.

2. Ask yourself if your hunger is being triggered by a familiar pattern, such as feeling bored, restless, or sad, or wanting a distraction. You now know some of your most common triggers, so see if any of them are involved.

3. Once you've identified a trigger, ask yourself if you really need to eat. Maybe you can find an alternative activity, one that simply postpones reacting to your trigger, such as:

Doing a household chore.
Calling a friend.

Checking your e-mails and answering some saved ones.
Reading a book.
Drinking a glass of water.

Any harmless diversion will do. Your goal is to insert a pause before you automatically react to a trigger. If you still feel hungry, go ahead and eat. But get in the habit of noticing your triggers this way—it's a basic step toward overcoming them and giving yourself more freedom to choose.

I promised myself one thing before addressing the problem of over-eating: The solution should work *here and now*. A great fault in dieting is that you make yourself unhappy today on the promise that you will be happier tomorrow. But desire doesn't work that way. "What am I hungry for?" exists in the present moment. The impulse you feel can be simplified into a few basic categories:

You're hungry for food.
You want to fill an emotional hole.
You want to fill a hole in your mind (such as low self-esteem, bad body image, or a sense of failure and frustration).
To these I would add a fourth impulse, which is spiritual. *You want to fill a hole in your soul.*

These are strong motivations, fueled by desire. Once you turn desire in the right direction, real transformation can take place. We all follow the path of desire every day. The impulse to get more out of life is natural and deep-seated. In this book we'll find out exactly what you're hungry for. Once you know, you will have a clear path that makes total sense in terms of mind, body, and spirit. Here's how you'll be transformed:

You will eat only when you are hungry for food.

You won't eat when what you're hungry for is emotional, in terms of comfort, security, love, bonding with others, or a feeling of joy.

You won't eat when what you are hungry for is a life that is relevant and meaningful, where you have a purpose and can meet your goals. These are needs of the mind.

You won't eat when what you're hungry for is spiritual, such as lightness of being or a higher vision of the soul.

Dieting: A False Escape

Some readers will say to themselves, "This all sounds well and good, but frankly, I just want to know what to eat and what not to eat." I know exactly how that goes. Crash diets offer the ultimate temptation, a quick fix. But look at what really happens:

Karen is an attractive middle-aged woman who stands in front of her mirror, frowning at what she sees. She wants to lose 10 pounds before her daughter's wedding, which is two weeks away, but Karen isn't discouraged. When she was twenty, she could lose 5 pounds over the weekend by going on a juice fast. If it worked then, it will work now.

And it does, almost. On her daughter's wedding day Karen has lost 7 pounds. She nearly starved to get there, but now she can celebrate. What she doesn't realize is that she's fallen into a trap. Her old eating habits will return soon, and so will the extra pounds. You can see her standing at the fridge the next day, as the following telegrams arrive at the mind-body connection:

Thank goodness the wedding's over. I can relax.
I worked hard. I deserve to treat myself.

Look at all the leftovers.

I can't starve myself forever.

I can't let this good food go to waste.

There is little chance, with these messages urging her on, that Karen will hold back from a nice big chunk of leftover wedding cake. Excuses come to mind every time you decide to overeat. The fact that Karen lost weight in a two-week sprint to the finish line means little compared to a lifetime of eating habits that keep adding extra pounds.

America is crazed over dieting. We'd all like to find a magic bullet that will solve years of bad habits. This has led to a bipolar condition in this country. At one extreme, McDonald's is the epitome of fatty, calorie-laden fast food, with 11 percent of all meals being eaten at chain restaurants, while at the other extreme most of the country is either on a diet or cheating on one. Crash dieting involves a voluntary form of amnesia. You forget what didn't work yesterday to plunge into the next gimmicky fad.

When you stand back, it's quite strange that people do exactly the opposite of what they know is good for them. But you can see it happening all around. Someone might say, "I'm trying to lose ten pounds," but then an hour later they reach for bread and butter in a restaurant as soon as they sit down and then end the meal with a warm brownie à la mode "just this once." A report from the Centers for Disease Control in 2013 found a small cutback in calories among schoolchildren—between 4 and 7 percent—but no weight loss, which was explained by a decrease in physical activity. Although American consumption of fast food fell by about 2 percent in the past decade, the people who were ranked as obese actually gained weight over the same period. One large online support group for people who have lost a large amount of weight takes the same "monkey on your back" approach as Alcoholics Anonymous. Overeating is a disorder that always threatens to return. Once you know that you are an overeater, you are resigned to living with cravings and must keep constant vigilance to avoid succumbing. Thus every calorie must be counted every day, and relapses are omens of impending loss of control. I am not judging this approach, but my intention is to find an alternative to the "monkey on your back."

What has worked for me is steady focus: I kept my eye on what I really wanted. First and foremost, I wanted to get back to normal, healthy eating—*and never slip again.* We all know that the second part is the real issue. Doctors call it noncompliance. The patient is told the right thing to do—eat a balanced diet with lots of fruits and vegetables, cut back on red meat, exercise regularly, give up smoking and excessive alcohol—but after a few days, weeks, or months, old habits are back in the saddle. Good advice about weight loss is everywhere, yet 70 percent of the adult population is either overweight or obese.

People aren't deliberately self-destructive. We don't follow good advice because, frankly, overeating makes us feel better than depriving ourselves or engaging in strenuous activity. A bucket of buttered popcorn triggers powerful, primitive brain mechanisms; the prospect of jogging three miles doesn't. Sharing dessert with your friends at a cozy restaurant feels convivial and comforting; running on a treadmill by yourself at the gym doesn't.

Dieters keep doing more of what never worked in the first place.

The slogan "Diets don't work" has been with us for decades, and it's absolutely true. Every long-term study has shown that less than 2 percent of dieters manage to lose a significant amount of weight (20 pounds or more) and keep it off for two years. We aren't a nation that totally lacks willpower. Failure is built into the whole diet scheme. What is a typical dieter's first impulse? To deprive themselves. They drastically cut their calorie intake. They fight against their cravings and vow to subsist on something like wheatgrass juice for a week. But all that deprivation creates another hole. Instead of feeling sad or lonely or unloved, you feel sad, lonely, unloved *and starving at the same time.*

I fully understand why people deprive themselves. A physical problem must require a physical solution. The extra pounds are visible every time you look in the mirror. The invisible holes aren't. Also, if overeating stands for lack of self-control, depriving yourself is a burst of super self-control. "I hate eating broccoli with lemon juice, but I'm forcing myself to." But added misery only compounds the problem. Keep in mind the classic moment in the movie *The Producers* when Zero Mostel can't calm down a gasping, panicky Gene Wilder.

"I'm hysterical! Once this starts I can't stop!" Wilder cries.

Not knowing what to do, Mostel throws a glass of water in his face. Wilder freezes in place.

"I'm hysterical! And now I'm wet!" he shrieks.

Still not knowing what to do, Mostel slaps him in the face.

Wilder wails, "I'm in pain! I'm wet! And I'm still hysterical!" A good reminder that making yourself feel worse never works. So pursue the next fad diet if you want to—you can even pursue it while you read this book, because once you see that fulfillment is better than depriving yourself, crash dieting will no longer be a temptation. The fact that weight loss can be connected with increasing happiness is the secret to why my approach works.

The Mind-Body Connection

To find out what you're hungry for, you must reconnect mind and body, looking beyond the simple circuitry we talked about before, which controls the basic hunger impulse through the hypothalamus. Because you can override simple signals from your body, even something as basic as hunger becomes involved in the whole brain. Not everybody has interfered with the natural setup that regulates appetite. We all know someone whose weight has never fluctuated since their late teens. They say things like the following:

My body tells me what it wants.
I feel uncomfortable if I gain 2 pounds.
I exercise because it feels so good.

These are statements rooted in the mind-body connection when it is working properly. Unfortunately, when it isn't working correctly, the mind-body connection short-circuits and bad habits tell the body what to do. The wrong signals are sent, and as the body reacts by getting fatter, more imbalanced, and ultimately sick, the mind ignores these signs of distress. Let's see why this happens.

Imagine that three telephone conversations converge at one

junction, which in reality is the meeting of three basic regions of the brain. Each region has something to tell you; each is sending neural messages to you at once. Each is seeking a different kind of satisfaction. The **lower brain** is satisfied when you feel good physically. The **limbic system** is satisfied when you feel good emotionally. The **higher brain** is satisfied when you are making good decisions for yourself.

The miracle of the human brain is that all three lines can merge and cooperate. The lower brain can send the message "I'm hungry," which the emotional brain accepts, because "Eating puts me in a good mood," so the higher brain can say, "Let's stop for a meal." This balancing act is natural, and it works to the benefit of all three regions of the brain. None of them must force its message through, trying to get heard by pushing the others out of the way.

Your brain is structured to find happiness at every level. For a baby, who operates almost totally with basic instincts from the lower brain, happiness means eating when he's hungry, sleeping when he's tired, being held when he's cold. But things become more complex when the other regions, the limbic system and the higher brain, start developing. Their version of happiness is far more complex.

As a young doctor, I knew these things medically but I wasn't paying attention personally. I look back at the dinner table and see a frustrated young man (with a patient young wife) whose brain was teeming with so much technical information (higher brain) that the inner voice, which cried out, "I'm unhappy and dissatisfied" (limbic system), got suppressed. At the same time, the most primitive voice in my head, which was afraid of failure and crashing under the pressure (reptilian brain), added disturbing background noise. No wonder meals passed by in a blur, offering a momentary flash of satisfaction. (I was fortunate to have been raised by loving parents, because at least my new family didn't fall apart as happened to so many young doctors I knew. I knew the value of giving and receiving love.)

You can't escape the three conversations going on in your mind all the time. Hundreds of choices are filtered through the higher brain every day, and each one carries an emotional coloring. This is uniquely human. If you put a pellet of food in front of a laboratory rat, it automatically eats it, and just as automatically the pleasure center in its brain lights up. But when you put food in front of a person, there can be any response imaginable. How often do people say things like the following?:

I'm too upset to eat.
I don't want this fish. I only like meat and potatoes.
I'm too busy right now.

Our brains have a pleasure center for food, just as a lab rat does, but our inner life is incredibly sophisticated. Emotions can override hunger or make it unnaturally strong. Distorted beliefs, arising in the higher brain, can interfere with both emotions and hunger—hence the anorexic teenager who sees a starved body in the mirror but feels "too fat" because of a warped mental image (I'm referring to one aspect of a complicated psychological and genetic disorder).

When you overeat, it may appear that the lower brain has run amok, forcing you into uncontrollable hunger. But the problem is actually systemic. Typically, it's a blend of impulse control (lower brain), trying to find comfort (emotional brain), and making bad choices (higher brain). All three are involved, forming a continuous dance.

This dance moves in a constant circle, as illustrated here:

Impulse
Emotion   **Choice**

Impulse: Your lower brain tells you if you're hungry, afraid, threatened, or aroused.

Emotion: Your limbic system tells you about your mood, positive or negative, and your emotional response in the present moment.

Choice: Your higher brain tells you that a decision must be made, leading to action.

At War with Herself

Let me illustrate how all of this works with a personal story. Tracy has had a weight problem since she was a teenager. She slid into several kinds of self-defeating behavior starting back then. She became defensive about her weight whenever her parents tried to talk about it. She developed a domineering personality, thinking that if she acted confident and bossy, no one would see how fragile she felt inside. When it came time to date boys, she quickly moved into sexual activity, because it was what boys wanted, and in turn she felt wanted. The more she acted out, though, the worse she felt about herself, so drugs and alcohol eventually followed.

All of that is well behind Tracy now. She is fifty and happily married, and she generally feels good about herself. But there's no getting around the fact that she is 80 to 100 pounds over her ideal weight. She was never my patient but a personal friend instead, and when we meet socially, it's usually at a restaurant. I don't judge how she eats or give advice, but at a typical meal, I've noticed a few things:

When she sits down, Tracy's first remark is usually that she's not hungry, but she'll find something to eat.

Waiting for the first course, she talks and eats several pieces of bread from the bread basket at the same time. She butters the bread without looking down at what she's doing.

She orders two courses, an appetizer and entrée, as soon as the server asks what she wants.

She always cleans her plate.

She never orders dessert but picks away at mine if I order one, generally eating at least half of it.

Looking at these habits, what strikes me is that Tracy acts them out unconsciously. She pays attention to me and our conversation but not to what her hands are doing. She's learned to blank out what she doesn't want to see. I'm sure that you now get what's going on here: Three areas of the brain are fighting a silent conflict, each using its own kind of message.

Tracy's lower brain keeps saying, "I'm hungry. More food. I'm still famished."

Her emotional brain keeps saying, "I don't feel good about myself. More food. I still feel bad."

Her higher brain keeps saying, "I know I shouldn't be eating like this. More food. Why bother resisting? It doesn't matter because the impulse will keep returning anyway."

It would be wonderful if somebody could take a snapshot of this cross talk in her brain, show it to Tracy, and make her see what's going on. Perhaps one day advanced brain scanning will do precisely that. But even with a perfect snapshot, the brain never stands still. Tracy's problem is always shifting. One minute she's obeying one part of her brain; the next minute another part takes charge. That's why in a single meal she can enjoy her food, hate herself for eating so much, promise to do better, and ignore the whole thing. Her behavior constantly contradicts itself.

This is the inner war being fought by everyone who struggles with their weight. Here's a secret: *You will never win this war.* If you could, you would have long ago. As long as you keep fighting with yourself, you will be stuck at the level of the problem. You must rise above the level of the problem and reach the level of the solution.

Tracy is following a typical and unfortunate pattern. Every hour of the day she obsesses about food, controlling her eating, and being overweight. She is mired at the level of the problem. What would it take to lift her to the level of the solution?

I assured her that the answer exists. "It's right inside you," I said. "When you obsess and worry, you are giving your brain the wrong assignment. You're telling it to send negative messages to every cell in your body. You can choose to stop doing that."

"But I feel bad," she protested. "I don't have any positive messages to send."

"No, not when you're so anxious and unhappy with yourself," I agreed. "But there's a positive message you've overlooked. Paying quiet attention to how your body feels is a powerful message, all by itself. Awareness isn't noisy or emotional. It looks on quietly, and that's the best state for your body to start rebalancing itself."

Tracy looked a bit mystified, but she smiled, because some part of her caught on. She was relieved that there was a way to get unstuck. Whenever anyone is trapped by habits, old conditioning, and out-of-control eating, they need to become quietly aware, without judgment, in a state that quiets the constant inner dialogue filling the mind. Awareness takes you from the level of the problem to the level of the solution.

Action Step:
The Basics of Awareness

So how do you go about increasing your awareness? Becoming more aware is easy and can be done anytime during the day using three basic techniques. They bring the three major regions of your brain into balance naturally and without effort.

Become **aware of your body.** Go inside and tune in to its physical sensations, whatever they are. Experience what your body is experiencing.

Become **aware of your emotions**. Close your eyes, put your attention on your heart, and see how you feel emotionally. Without getting involved, be centered and observe these feelings.

Become **aware of your choices**. Find a time when you are calm, maybe early in the morning upon waking or while you are relaxing in the shower, and examine the best way to make the decisions you are facing. The best decision making comes from an inner state of restful alertness.

I experienced a real transformation by adopting these basic techniques, which take only a moment to practice. I hadn't realized something quite fundamental about my mind. It's a perpetual motion machine. Given a chance, it runs all the time, piling up thought after thought, emotion after emotion. I wasn't giving it time to do some important things. It needed to calm down, to reflect upon the moment, to consider how I felt, to ask my body how it felt. "How are we doing?" is such a simple question—the *we* including body, emotions, and intellect—and yet most of us don't ask it often enough. Asking a friend "How are you doing?" is a reassuring thing to do. You deserve the same if you want your body to be your friend.

Try these techniques out for yourself, with no expectations or prejudgment. Being in tune isn't difficult, but many overweight people have gotten out of touch with their bodies because when you get right down to it they don't like themselves anymore. They are reluctant to look at their emotions, because they worry about what they might find. They feel trapped by bad choices in the past, which makes it harder to look afresh at new possibilities. All of this can be overcome by weaning your brain away from its old conditioning. There's no need to struggle. Just make these new techniques into a habit and allow change to arrive naturally.

A Success Story

Dana is a success story of the mind-body approach, and she illustrates what I mean by an effortless way to lose weight. What's so important is how she reached her turning point. Here is her story:

"I maintained my college weight for years," Dana recounts. "In my thirties I changed jobs and landed in a company that provided on-site meals. I got into the habit of popping downstairs for lunch, and most of the time I was either thinking about my job or talking to a co-worker while we ate. I didn't walk outside enough, and if something looked really good in the cafeteria, I ate it without thinking."

Without really noticing it, Dana gained 15 pounds over one winter, which shocked her. She began dieting to get the weight off but found it hard to stay motivated. Assuming that all it took was more willpower, she kept promising herself that she would take charge of her appetite, but somehow that day never came. Instead, her stress level rose.

"I left the company and started a small business, just as the downturn came. The business stalled, and then I ran short of money. I began doing something I had never done before. Every afternoon I had a big Snickers bar washed down with half a can of diet soda. Frankly, I didn't even think about my weight. I was too anxious all the time."

Eventually her business troubles reversed, which was good news. But none of her old clothes fit anymore, and when Dana looked in the mirror, she felt frustrated and disappointed in herself.

A crash diet took off about half the weight she needed to lose, but by the time I saw Dana, most of it had returned. Ironically, the fact that she was getting new clients in her consulting business fueled the problem. There were more lunches eaten out with clients, more hours spent on the phone, more days when she arrived home exhausted after six at night.

It took a mind-body approach to change these negative trends. I proposed that she do the three things we covered earlier: feel her body, observe her emotions, and make more-aware choices.

My aim was to get Dana to tune in, because her story is about losing the connection between mind, body, and emotions. This new approach intrigued her, especially when I assured her that it was effortless—the only demand was for moments of paying attention, which was an expenditure of time that she could easily afford.

"At first it was strange to watch myself," she said. "I began to catch myself thoughtlessly buttering a roll in a restaurant, so I'd stop, and when I tuned in, I found that I wasn't actually hungry. The message was right there in front of me. All I had to do was feel it."

Now, a year later, she is back down to her college weight, but more important, Dana has learned the power of paying attention. Awareness is the key to weight loss, once you train yourself to notice the natural signals present in the body at any moment. It takes time and repetition to cause long-term imbalances to shift, but they will. You are the choice-maker who can create any change you desire.

A Doctor's Perspective

Like every other young doctor in the seventies, I came of age in medicine knowing absolutely zero about the mind-body connection. My medical specialty was endocrinology, the field that deals with hormones. As a young doctor I was fascinated with how the tiniest secretion of chemicals could make someone afraid, courageous, angry, sexually aroused, or hungry in a matter of seconds. The secret to Dr. Jekyll becoming Mr. Hyde lies in a molecule! That discovery sparked my imagination, and I originally thought I'd be content to stay in the laboratory examining the effects of hormones, because their action and interaction is astonishingly complex.

But when I went into private practice, I saw the devastating effect of hormones firsthand. Stress hormones were culprits in disorders that could ruin people's lives, often in cruel social ways. "He's lazy and dull" is the stigma attached too often to thyroid deficiency. Soldiers have been anxious about seeming to be cowards for centuries, but another hormone, adrenaline, leads to flight as much as fight. In addition, when the adrenaline rush is over, the body is physically depleted. Expose a soldier to enough situations where fight-or-flight is triggered, and the result is shell shock. Countless combatants have accused themselves of being cowards—and were stigmatized by fellow soldiers—because they were simply exhausted at the hormonal level. This stigma didn't begin to fade until it was realized that every soldier will become shell-shocked given enough time at the front lines. No moral failing is involved; the stigma was incredibly unfair.

My experience in private practice was more everyday but just as much about stigmas. Many of the patients I saw—literally thousands—were overweight women who felt ashamed and hoped that they had a "gland problem" instead of some personal flaw. It was discouraging when I told 99 percent of them that their hormonal levels were normal. They went away sad, discouraged, and sometimes hopeless. Many had to fight against their own shame and guilt simply to go to a doctor and ask for help. What I left them with was worse than what they came in with. That was unacceptable to me; I began searching for a missing link. Starting in the late eighties, I saw that a body problem was actually a mind-body problem, and it wasn't long before another dimension appeared. What my patients—and countless more people—had was a mind-body-spirit problem.

For me the breakthrough in seeing medical problems as mind-body-spirit problems was exciting and productive. I learned how good it felt to be centered and relaxed, to feel comfortable within myself all the time. You value something more when you know you can reach it. Empty dreams are lulling, but once you find that mind-body-spirit is real, nothing is more enticing. At last you get to fulfill your deepest yearnings. The secret is revealed: *Life is about fulfillment.*

Once this secret is no longer hidden, everything changes. You see with sudden clarity that all kinds of things aren't fulfilling. Some are distractions, like having a martini at five o'clock or getting hooked on video games. Some are obstacles, like ignoring your negative feelings and letting them fester. It feels good to think you have no issues with anger, fear, guilt, and shame, but your body can't be fooled. It feels everything you try so desperately to avoid.

I had no deeper wish than to show others the way out. Years of sending away patients to feel discouraged and frustrated needed to be turned around. For people who struggle with their weight, the body they see in the mirror is a mask. Behind it lie bad habits, distorted beliefs, low expectations, and every variety of discouragement. The cruelest form of starvation is to tie someone up and put a banquet before them, inches out of reach. Fulfillment is such a banquet, and for countless people it is being held out of reach. They are starved for fulfillment and don't know why they can't reach it.

Getting a fulfilling life isn't as easy as watching the Super Bowl with a plate of nachos in your lap or enjoying a nice lunch with a friend while the waiter brings an extra dessert fork "just in case." But I promise you that the journey to fulfillment is the most excit-ing project you could possibly undertake. Let's be companions in the spirit of hope, trust, and joy.

Making It Personal:
A Commitment, Just Between Us

There's much more to say in the following pages, but now you know where our journey is taking us—toward a holistic solution. I'd like you to pause here and make a commitment. It's your side of a silent contract between us.

Your side: You agree to follow the mind-body program outlined in the following pages for 30 days. You will not go on a diet. You will not indulge in negative judgments against your body. You will live in the present and disregard the old conditioning that has led only to frustration and disappointment. With an open mind, you will focus on walking the path of fulfillment.

My side: I agree to guide you to holistic change, giving you tested principles and action steps that have proven effective at the Chopra Center for years. Together, you and I are going to get your brain's messages back into balance by giving you what you really want. Fulfillment must exist physically, emotionally, and mentally. You'll know how to measure your success on each level.

Body: Your body will feel lighter, more energetic, and increasingly vital.

Emotions: Your mood will be happier, more uplifting, and increasingly positive.

Mind: Your decisions and choices will add to your vision of a better life and make the vision come true.

Your brain is meant to take care of you, which is what its amazing complexity is designed for. The mind-body approach fills an aching gap in every program for weight loss that I've encountered. The pounds always come back after they're lost because what needed to change—the person who uses food to fill invisible holes—remains the same. Here is a chance to transform yourself. When that happens you'll see a change not only in the way you look but in the way you work at your job, the way you see your surroundings, and the way you love the people in your life, including yourself.

PART ONE

THE CHOPRA SOLUTION

Change Your Story,
Change Your Body

Power Points

- You are writing your own life story. Your body is a physical projection of your story.
- Your story consists of your experiences and how you process them, physically and mentally.
- If you are overweight, your story probably reflects negative themes about food, eating, and body image.
- Before you change your story, you should know some facts about the mind-body connection. Knowledge is power.
- To activate the mind-body connection, state your conscious goals to yourself. This is the most powerful message you can send to your body.

At this moment you and I, even though we're complete strangers, are doing the same thing. We are living out our life stories. The biggest part of everyone's story could be titled "How I Make Myself Happy." Every story contains the same goal, because even if person A is playing professional football in order to reach the Super Bowl, person B is commuting to work every day, and person C is raising two small children at home, those differences disappear before the overriding aim to be happy as best we can.

You can change your story so that one chapter will read, "How I Lost All the Weight I Wanted To (and Kept It Off, Thank You)." Now, every story has themes that run through it, and presently your themes around food and eating are probably negative. When I talk to overweight patients, the same themes repeat themselves, often for decades. Any of this sound familiar?

- "I've tried everything and read all kinds of diet books, but nothing has worked. I might as well give up."
- "I must be genetically programmed to be overweight."
- "I'm unattractive anyway. My appearance makes me miserable."
- "I'm too old to start all over again."
- "This is my body, and I have to live with it."
- "I know I should exercise, but I can't stay motivated."
- "I know the right foods to eat, but I give in to temptations and cravings."
- "It's all just too hard."

When most doctors hear such remarks, they aren't paying attention to the psychological implications—the doctor is trying to isolate a physical complaint. Beyond that, most physicians, including myself, received no training in nutrition when they were in medical school, only the most basic training about weight (covered in lectures on endocrinology), and spent almost zero hours studying the effects of dieting. As for emotions, those require a psychiatrist or other therapist. They aren't part of a typical physician's job description.

It's incomplete medicine when the mind-body connection is being ignored. In anyone's story, the main themes aren't incidental or irrelevant. When you feed negative input into the brain, it changes, shaping itself to conform to the messages it receives. The brain has no mind of its own. It cannot choose which instructions to obey and which to ignore. You are the one who possesses a mind, and you are the author writing your story. Which means that you have the most control. You can feed negative messages to your brain or positive messages—the choice is yours.

I realize that neuroscience treats the brain and the mind as one and the same. That's because the mind is invisible, while the brain is a semisolid object that can be touched and measured. My position is different and I think closer to real life. The brain is like a radio receiving what the mind has to say. When you hear a concert broadcast, you don't mistake the radio for Mozart. If someone whispers "I love you" into your ear, you are the one who falls in love, not your limbic system. The mind comes first because the person comes first.

Your body is the physical record of your life story as you've lived it until today. Every pound represents a choice to eat a certain way, and each bite is silently influenced by a set of habits, a list of likes and dislikes, and how others around you are eating. If you are unhappy with your weight, those extra pounds are likely to represent some unhappy experiences: moments of frustration, high levels of stress, anxiety over a job or a relationship. If your body represents your story so far, the natural way to change your body is to change your story.

In my experience, when someone is overweight, they say negative things to themselves over and over. Remember, when you change your internal messages, you aren't just talking to yourself. You are writing new pages in the book of your life. The key is to change the negative messages so that instead of reinforcing bad behaviors, you begin to reinforce good ones.

Action Step:
Reverse the Messages.

When you feel unfulfilled, you can't fool yourself into feeling satisfied. But you can reverse the negative messages that make you feel stuck. Unhappiness thrives on inertia—it's easy to keep feeling the same way today as you felt yesterday. The brain supports inertia unless you give it something new to process.

So let's start doing that. Whenever the familiar themes voiced by overweight people come to mind, stop and notice what you're thinking. Then substitute a counterthought, a positive antidote. In this way, you jump-start the process of rewriting your story and changing your body as you do.

In the following list, the positive messages are just suggestions. Feel free to invent your own new messages. That's the best way to really take control of the input your brain is receiving.

1. *Negative:* "I've tried everything and read all kinds of diet books, but nothing has worked. I might as well give up."

Positive: "Today's a new day. Whatever happened in the past doesn't count. There's always a solution."

2. *Negative:* "I must be genetically programmed to be overweight."

Positive: "I can't change my genes, but I can trigger other genes that regulate normal appetite. Anyway, I know there are people who have lost huge amounts of weight. Their genes didn't hold them back, and mine won't either."

3. *Negative:* "I'm unattractive anyway. My appearance makes me miserable."

Positive: "The ugly duckling was miserable, too, until he amazed everyone by becoming beautiful. I'm going to be like that. I already have beautiful aspects that others appreciate. I'm going to accentuate those qualities with a body to match."

4. Negative: "I'm too old to start all over again."

Positive: "Age doesn't matter, because when I lose weight, I am going back in time. I'm reversing the aging process to get back to where my body used to be—and wants to be."

5. Negative: "This is my body, and I have to live with it."

Positive: "Every cell in my body is being renewed all the time. I don't have the same body today that I had a year ago. So if I am always renewing my body, I can renew it to be better."

6. Negative: "I know I should exercise, but I can't stay motivated."

Positive: "I don't need to exercise if that's too hard right now. All I need to do is move, and there are lots of ways I can do that. Some, like dancing or doing simple yoga, are even fun. Once I remember how good it feels to walk and move around, motivation won't be a problem."

7. Negative: "I know the right foods to eat, but I give in to temptations and cravings."

Positive: "Cravings mean that my body wants to be satisfied. I will give it what it wants by tuning in and listening. I'd like to be fulfilled, and food isn't the only way to get there. The happier I make myself, the less I will use food as a crutch."

8. Negative: "It's all just too hard."

Positive: "The hard part was deprivation, discipline, and struggling against hunger. I'm not going to do any of those things anymore. Finding satisfaction is easy, and it's my new path."

Substituting new thoughts is really a kind of brain therapy, using the higher brain's capacity for belief. Thinking is a complex business, but beliefs gain their power by attaching themselves to emotions. It's now well known that memories stick with us largely because we invest in them emotionally. Everything from your first kiss to being told off by your first-grade teacher can stay with you for years, while events that have no emotional value quickly fade. (Can you remember the first time you brushed your teeth or made your bed? The first bottle of detergent you bought or how many times you parked your car last week?)

The belief system of overweight people can be tagged with words that are loaded with emotion: *fatty, loser, failure, lazy, greedy, sloppy, gluttonous, ugly,* and so on. We need to alter these loaded terms with new ones that are equally emotional yet positive. Feeling good requires your brain to fill specific receptors with chemical messages. If these receptors get overloaded positively, food won't give you the fix it once did—this is just like drug addicts whose receptors for pain and pleasure are so overloaded that they must take more and more of their drug to get even a small fix. If you keep eating all day, your brain response gets dulled. The natural balance of hunger and satiation is thrown off. Basically, you are throwing damp logs on the fire. The fuel is right, but it won't catch fire.

Nourished on Every Level

Let me introduce words that carry positive emotional coloring: *light, vital, success, winner, satisfied, buoyant, renewed, free.* When you feed them into your brain, you reinforce new pathways that affect every cell in your body. Thanks to the mind-body connection, which is holistic, each word influences you as a complete person. Every level of our life gets nourished. In fact, *nourished* is the best single term to describe how you are going to change your life story. No doubt you already see why. Food satisfies our need to feel nourished; it's the opposite of deprivation. Being complex creatures, we associate food with all kinds of related experiences: home, mother, childhood, family, togetherness, warmth, protection, abundance, giving.

These are powerful tags for powerful experiences. When you mix them with negative experiences that are also powerful, the good gets polluted. I'm not suggesting that your story should be all sweetness and light; feeding your brain with propaganda is wrong and pointless. In everyone's life those potent tags—mother, home, family, childhood—carry memories of hurt and sorrow, too. But reality is always renewing itself. You can and should inject fresh messages if you want to move forward in your life. There is no reason to be the prisoner of old conditioning and negative memories.

Action Step:
Nourished by "Light"

You can prove to yourself how nourishing a new word can be once it begins to be your personal theme. Let's use the word *light*. Since it's the opposite of *heavy*, this word is one of the best for our purposes. The more you bring *light* into your life, the easier it will be to lose weight. Why? Because *light* covers so many positive experiences. Look at the following usages:

Lighthearted
Light-handed
Enlightened
Feeling light and bright

The light of inspiration
Lightness of being
The light of the soul
The light of God

If you had these things in your life, it would be much easier for your body to be light. Your mind would be sending messages that are the opposite of *heavy, dull, inert, tired, bored, dark, unenlightened*. Start to rid yourself of those messages and let your body conform to *lightness* and all of its positive connotations.

With this background, you can proceed to use *light* in various ways, beginning with the physical sensation of being light.

Exercise: *Filling with Light*

Sit in a quiet room by yourself. Close your eyes and take a few deep breaths until you feel centered and ready. (It's best to sit upright if you can rather than lounging back in your chair.)

Breathing normally, visualize light filling your chest each time you inhale. The light is soft, warm, and white. Watch it suffuse your chest. Now exhale normally, but leave the light inside.

On your next breath, take in more light. See the light filling your chest now begin to suffuse the rest of your body, moving down into your abdomen. Don't force the visualization, and don't worry if you have trouble seeing the light—even a faint sense of white light is good enough.

With each breath, let the light suffuse your arms, then your hands all the way to the fingertips. Let it suffuse your legs down to your toes. Finally, send the light into your head and out the top in a beam that reaches high.

Sit with the light for a few moments, then lift your arms, letting them float upward as if the light is causing them to rise. You are like a balloon filled completely with light. Enjoy the sensation, then open your eyes.

This is a good exercise to counteract feelings of dullness, heaviness, fatigue, and sadness. The sensation of being physically light, paired with the visualization of inner light, creates a big change in how you relate to your body. But there's much more that you can do with the theme of light:

- Favor lighter foods, the fresher and more natural the better.
- Drink lighter beverages—flavored spring water instead of sodas, for example, or alcohol-free beer.
- Do one thing every day that makes you feel lighthearted.
- Be gentler with yourself and others, using a lighter hand.
- Wear lighter colors and lighter fabrics.
- When you feel happy, let your light shine so others can see it.
- Be in the light by associating with people who inspire you.
- Read inspiring poetry and spiritual literature, gaining nourishment at the level of the soul.

Once you get it—that *light* nourishes at every level—this is a wonderful theme to play with. Each meaning of a single word can be turned into countless actions. A life that is lived in the light is the best anyone could ask for.

Since every life story is complex, there's a need for simplicity so that you can change without getting lost in the weeds—and let's face it, everyday existence gets pretty weedy, filled with distractions, complications, accidents, and obstacles. Anyone can benefit by using the simple model of themes or tags. If you devoted yourself to just two themes we've been discussing—*light* and *nourishing*—your existence would be totally transformed.

Getting the Message

Let's go deeper into the mind-body connection. The words in your head follow a circular path known as a feedback loop.

You have a thought.
It registers in your brain.
The brain sends chemical signals to every cell in your body.
The cells react and send a message back to the brain.

As feedback runs through the loop, you experience a new sensation, emotion, or thought. Some aspects go unnoticed, however, which is why it took decades before modern medicine discovered that every mental event affects the body, too. The research to discover the brain's microscopic, fleeting neurotransmitters—the carriers of messages from cell to cell—was quite painstaking.

Changing negative input to positive input makes a world of difference. A few basic principles apply to everyone (assuming the absence of serious physical or mental disorders). We've been discussing them already, but it's good to be specific.

Principle #1: To change your body, first change your story.
Principle #2: Every story is about how to be happy.
Principle #3: If you find a better way to be happy than by overeating, your body will naturally return to its balanced state.

If you are chronically overweight, one or more of these basic principles needs your attention. You are the author of your own story. Let me give an example of how the plot can go out of control, even though it doesn't have to.

Jerry is forty-five and securely employed. He went through a rough divorce this year. Now it's ten months later, and Jerry must have started to find comfort in overeating, because he can squeeze the beginning of an inner tube around his waist. But this doesn't worry him; he's not in the market for a new relationship yet. He can afford to let himself go a little; it's one of the perks of being a bachelor again.

A month later Jerry goes to the doctor for a routine physical. He tells the nurse she's made a mistake when she weighs him at 20 pounds heavier than the year before. But the scale is right, and Jerry's doctor notices a rise in blood pressure and what he calls "prediabetic" blood sugar. Something needs to be done. Jerry immediately joins a gym. He cuts out frozen pizza, a mainstay of his diet since his wife left him, but in the end, he works too hard to get to the gym more than once or twice a week. He starts dating a woman who has no problem, she says, with his extra weight. She's been gaining some herself, and although Jerry isn't too pleased with the medical side of things, the two happily indulge in going to expensive restaurants. A series of tiny rationalizations starts to accumulate in his mind:

I look good for my age, and I feel good.
I've had a rough time. I can let myself go a little.
I never liked being nagged about my weight.
I'm an adult. I can eat what I want.
There are lots of people heavier than I am.

There is no villain in this story, only a steady stream of thoughts and feelings that gradually produce a bad result. And while all of this was happening to Jerry, the mind-body feedback loop was always paying attention.

Your mind has tremendous power, so as you begin to change your story, you need to know some guidelines:

1. You are not your body. You are the creator of your body.
2. You have created your present body using both conscious and unconscious thoughts.
3. You can create a new body through conscious choices.
4. Your body is a verb (a process), not a noun (a fixed object).
5. You continually recycle your material body—almost all of it— once a year (stomach lining every five days; skin once a month; skeleton every three months; liver every six weeks; genetic material every six weeks).
6. You constantly change the activity of your genes by the same signals sent by thoughts, emotions, and behavior.

Because they see themselves in the mirror as a solid object standing alone in space, people don't grasp that the body isn't a thing at all. It is an ever-shifting process. Imagine a building that looks like any other except that when you get closer, you see that the bricks are flying out of place and renewed with fresh bricks all the time. That's your body. Even though your skeleton seems solid, for example, it exchanges calcium constantly with the rest of the body, and as these atoms move, their replacements respond to change. A marathon runner's skeleton looks totally different when examined at the cellular level from that of someone who is totally sedentary. Even wearing a new pair of shoes is enough to change the shape of your leg bones. When you were twenty, your upper leg was composed of twice as much muscle as fat. In the absence of physical activity, there will be twice as much fat as muscle when you turn fifty or sixty.

Even though your organs hold basically the same shape, they are constantly exchanging their fundamental building blocks. That's why I like to say that the body is a verb, not a noun. People are surprised to discover that this extends down to their genes. You can't add or lose the genes you were born with, but genes aren't fixed; they are switched on and off by many factors. Dr. Dean Ornish and his Harvard colleagues have shown that up to five hundred genes change their output when a person makes positive lifestyle changes, such as improved diet, moderate exercise, meditation, and stress management.

The Biggest Obstacle: Mixed Messages

If the mind has so much power, why do people feel powerless when they want to change? It's a question of mixed messages being processed at the mind-body connection. Every overeater knows what it's like to fight against food cravings and have the cravings win. That's a perfect example of two messages clashing: one saying, "I mustn't give in," the other saying, "I can't help myself."

If you could take a freeze-frame picture of your mind as you reach for a tempting snack, the choice between "Eat this" and "Don't eat this" should be simple to understand. Your story for that moment would read, "She wasn't really hungry, so she ate a carrot stick instead of a candy bar." Such simplicity doesn't always exist in real life, however. In fact, it almost never does. All kinds of mental events are taking place at once. Imagine that six telegrams are arriving at the same time, which might read something like this:

I'm in a rush, no time for a real meal.
I'm feeling restless.
Sugar makes me feel good.
I can't worry about nutrition at this moment.
The candy machine is right here.
I wish I could stop myself.

All six telegrams arrive at the same place together. What happens next is that you make a choice. What will it be? Most adults know that the rational choice—in terms of health, weight, nutrition, and overall satisfaction—is to walk past the candy machine. But five of the six telegrams urge you to eat instead; only one is clear and rational. The snack food industry makes a fortune by counting on you to ignore reason and give in to your impulses, forgetting what's good for you and grabbing a candy bar on the run.

The irony, as millions of people pack empty, sugary food into their bodies, is that you and you alone have control over the mind-body connection. The words *yes* and *no* are not foreign to you, and you know how to weigh the pros and cons of the decisions you make. Your whole life is spent making choices. But the mind-body connection goes wrong for one simple reason. The six telegrams bring messages that fight against each other. This leads to a state, only recently discovered by neuroscience, known as *cross-inhibition*. It's a bit of jargon that explains the conflicting messages in our heads. Everyone who struggles with their weight knows how the fight generally runs:

"I shouldn't give in" versus "I'm going to anyway."
"This isn't good for me" versus "But it tastes so good."
"I can't let myself down this way" versus "So what? You do it all the time."

Cross-Inhibition: Who's Going to Win?

The messages in our heads do more than just speak to us. They try to defeat the other messages. This happens quite literally, as advanced brain research has revealed. The group of neurons that sends out one message ("Don't reach for that ice cream bar") emits chemical signals to block the opposite message being sent by another group of neurons ("Go ahead. Eat that ice cream bar"). In this regard, your brain is acting like some trees, such as redwoods and black walnuts, whose roots secrete chemicals that prevent other trees from sprouting nearby. Only in this case, the defeating chemicals come from both sides. A choice must be made, however, and your brain is wired so that one message will win out in the end; otherwise you'd be in a constant state of indecision.

Cross-inhibition is good—if the winning message is the right one. Your brain is incredibly efficient at reducing complex decisions to yes or no. Think of all the elements that go into deciding what college to attend or whom to marry or whether to have a baby. It would be unbearable to live in perpetual indecision. Your brain is set up to lead you to make a choice, but what is even more fascinating, once *yes* defeats *no*, your decision feels final. Usually it also feels good and right.

But sometimes the bad messages are unfairly weighted against the good ones, and then trouble starts. Your choices don't sit right. You get the eater's equivalent of buyer's remorse ("I can't believe I ate the whole thing"). What makes the impulse to overeat so much stronger than the impulse not to? It's not hunger per se. The mind-body connection tells a different story. Bad messages have become unfairly weighted through repetition that changes the brain in favor of giving in.

Why Bad Messages Win

1. Habit.
2. A history of wrong choices.
3. Sense of failure.
4. Lack of impulse control.
5. Family and peer pressure.

You may not remember all the times that these bad messages won out over good messages, but your body does, thanks to well-worn pathways in the brain.

Overeaters Anonymous and other support groups try to push the balance the other way. A personal sponsor or group buddy can be telephoned, and that person reinforces the good messages that need to come through. They are the reverse of the bad ones. What feels like moral reinforcement is actually a tactic to alter the brain's hardwiring.

When Good Messages Win

1. You find a way to break a bad habit.
2. You lay down a pattern of right choices.
3. You gain a sense of success.
4. You have impulse control.
5. Family and peer pressure don't influence you to overeat just to go along.

These two lists point to a valuable conclusion. We get fat because the messages that lead to overeating have been defeating the messages that say, "You don't have to eat this." (Careful monitoring supports this conclusion. When overweight people are told to write down everything they eat during the day, almost all are consuming more calories than they think they are.) After enough defeats, the "eat" message has worn a groove in the brain, and this bit of hardwiring ensures that future food cravings will be triumphant.

By the same token, if you build up victories over the "eat" messages, a state of balance is restored. New pathways form in the brain. When the hunger impulse arises, the contest will be more equal, and over time food cravings will disappear. At that point, the mind-body connection will be healthy again. Proper weight will be maintained automatically.

What you should take away from our discussion of cross-inhibition is two lessons:

1. Conflicting messages try to defeat each other in the brain.

2. The more you listen to the good messages, the easier it is for them to defeat the bad messages.

Action Step:
Choose a Better Message.

When you feel the impulse to eat outside mealtime, that's a message from your brain. Impulses are quick and powerful messages, which is why it's almost impossible to control them on the spot. Instead of fighting your hunger impulse, a better way is to let the rest of your brain catch up. The decision-making part is slower to react, but if you retrain your brain, decision making becomes better and better, while impulses are brought back into balance.

The next time you feel a food craving, use the technique of S-T-O-P:

S = Stop what you're doing.

T = Take a 1-minute breathing break. As you inhale and exhale, count to 20, as follows: 1 on the inhale, 2 on the exhale, 3 on the inhale, and so on.

O = Observe the bodily sensation of hunger. Rate it from 1 to 5, with 5 standing for "famished" and 1 standing for "not really hungry."

P = Proceed with awareness.

The whole point of this technique is to get you to "Proceed with awareness," because that indicates that your higher brain is now part of your inner conversation. Proceeding with awareness means you decide what to do next, which is far better than robotically obeying the lower brain's hunger impulse if it has gotten out of balance.

What kind of aware choice can you make now? Here are some suggestions:

- Drink a full glass of water. You will satisfy an urge to feel full, and water suppresses appetite.
- Eat ten almonds or a slice of whole-wheat bread or five crackers. A small ingestion of 100 to 200 calories acts to suppress hunger for 1 to 2 hours afterward (a study in which college students were asked to eat a slice of whole-wheat bread before every meal found that they lost a significant amount of weight doing nothing else).
- Read an interesting book or article for ten minutes, then check in to see if you are still hungry.

In my own life, the trick of eating ten nuts when I feel a craving has been quite effective, by the way. Sometimes the simplest choices work out the best.

If you make a choice that leads you to avoid a craving, be sure to stop and appreciate your small victory. "I did the right thing—good for me" is a powerful message when repeated many times over the course of weeks and months, because it reinforces choice making over giving in to cravings.

This action step makes you conscious of what you're doing, and losing weight is all about conscious choices. As with smokers who give up their nicotine habit, repetition is the key. The more times you try to quit, the higher your odds for success. That's why the people who successfully kick cigarettes are the ones who have attempted to repeatedly—as often as they backslide. Eventually the decision to resist their craving wins out. Repetition brings reinforcement, bit by bit. The same holds true for deciding not to overeat.

Making It Personal:
Themes for the Week

This chapter has given you ways to change your story, including the powerful tool of introducing the themes of *light* and *nourish* into your life. There are other themes that work just as well. If this approach excites you, why not focus on a different theme for every day of the week? There are countless ways you can replace an old theme with a new one that is more positive and stimulating to mind and body.

Monday: Turn *passive* into *active*.

Tuesday: Turn *dull* into *vibrant*.

Wednesday: Turn *routine* into *surprising*.

Thursday: Turn *stale* into *fresh*.

Friday: Turn *pessimistic* into *optimistic*.

Saturday: Turn *work* into *recreation*.

Sunday: Turn *ordinary* into *inspiring*.

Here are some specific suggestions to get you started; once you do, new possibilities will quickly come to mind.

Monday: Turning *passive* into *active*.

Take any passive activity that occurs during the day—watching TV would top most people's list—and substitute an activity, like a stroll around the block. Instead of riding the elevator, take the stairs. Instead of letting others do all the talking, change the conversation to something you're interested in. As you do any of these things, reinforce the message in your mind: "Now I'm being active."

Tuesday: Turning *dull* into *vibrant*.

Define *vibrant* any way you choose: a bright color, a spicy taste, a sparkling conversation. Today, inject the vibrancy into your routine. Wear a brighter color, eat spicier or more colorful food. Look at rainbows on YouTube or stand by a fountain in the sunlight. As you do any of these things, reinforce the message in your mind: "Now I'm being vibrant."

Wednesday: Turning **routine** into **surprising**.

Life is made comfortable by following a routine, but existence would be dull without a dash of excitement. Today, change some part of your routine. Go to an exciting new restaurant or find an exciting new shop. Instead of reading *USA Today* as you ride the train to work, why not read something inspirational? Excite someone you love with a note of adoration. In your intimate relationship, dare to suggest something exciting in bed—share a fantasy or explore a new sensation of pleasure. As you do any of these things, reinforce the message in your mind: "Now I'm being exciting."

Thursday: Turning **stale** into **fresh**.

Every theme has a broad meaning, and with *freshness* you can look almost anywhere. Today, throw out all the stale food in your refrigerator and bring in fresh fruits and vegetables. Put fresh flowers on the table. Notice something fresh about an old friend and tell it to her in an appreciative way. As you do any of these things, reinforce the message in your mind: "Now I'm bringing in some freshness."

Friday: Turning **pessimistic** into **optimistic**.

It's all too easy to get into the rut of bemoaning the state of the world. Today, take any pessimistic attitude and explore how to take an optimistic angle. Think in terms of hope, new possibilities, the goodness in people, the healing brought by time. Find a way to sympathize with those who are suffering rather than blaming them for their situation. Look at your own future the same way, dwelling on things that are going to get better. As you do any of these things, reinforce the message in your mind: "Now I'm being optimistic."

Saturday: Turning **work** into **recreation**.

The weekend is for play and relaxation, but too often we find ourselves still working, either around the house or with extra work from the job. Today, find a way to enjoy recreation, and make it true "re-creation." Participate in an activity that makes you feel renewed. Plant a tree, spend time with children drawing pictures on a sidewalk, explore a nearby woods, get up early and watch the sunrise. As you do any of these things, reinforce the message in your mind: "Now I'm re-creating myself."

Sunday: Turning **ordinary** into **inspiring**.

One day of the week should be extraordinary, and nothing is more extraordinary than connecting with your highest vision. Today, read inspirational scripture or poetry. Look at great art, listen to masterpieces of music—whatever it is that nourishes your soul. As you do any of these things, reinforce the message in your mind: "Now I'm feeling inspired."

Purity, Energy, and Balance

Power Points

- An ideal diet follows three themes: purity, energy, and balance.
- Purity is about removing toxins and returning to nature.
- Energy is about more than fueling your body—a higher kind of energy comes from the joy of eating.
- Balance is about your body adapting to the life you want to live.

---

n my own life, I found a way to live the story I wanted to live. We've already covered one theme, *light*, that became central for me. It still is. I don't just eat lighter. I aim to lighten my burden of stress and avoid adding to anyone else's burden. For thirty years I've delved into what the word *enlightenment* means and how to achieve it. It's wonderful how themes can change a story in so many dimensions. They affect everything: mind, body, emotions, and spirit.

I hope you've experienced the benefits of lightness, beginning with adding more salads, more fruits and vegetables, and smaller portions. But the total benefit doesn't arrive until you begin to treat a theme holistically. By adding three new themes in this chapter, we can move closer to an ideal diet, and, far more important, you will have a deeper sense of the story you want to live. The new themes are:

Purity
Energy
Balance

These are familiar terms, and one of the encouraging trends in American eating is that people are putting more value on a diet that contains pure—that is, natural—foods. But there's also a backlash effect that discourages compliance. "This is how I should eat" lowers motivation more often than it raises it. "This is how I enjoy eating" needs no finger-wagging; we go there automatically. My goal is to help you prefer a diet that is pure, energetic, and balanced because you enjoy it more than any other kind.

Purity

The accumulation of toxins
in the body/mind system
leads to uncontrolled weight gain, accelerated aging,
and impaired physical functions.
Eliminating toxins awakens the body's
capacity for renewal and returning to natural balance.
Toxins need to be eliminated from body, mind, and soul.

The preceding passage summarizes the overall goal of *purity* as a theme in your life. The opposite of *pure* is *impure*, *toxic*, *polluted*, *adulterated*, and so on. There is much to say about eliminating toxic feelings and relationships. Every theme works best when you apply it holistically. Here we focus mainly on food as a starting point.

Do:

- As mentioned earlier, throw out all old, stale food.
- Minimize processed foods.
- Keep fruits and vegetables as fresh as possible when storing.
- Prefer whole grains and natural sweeteners.
- Eliminate hydrogenated and trans fats.
- Buy organic produce (if affordable).
- Favor deeply green vegetables like spinach and kale, along with the rest of the cabbage family (including broccoli and cauliflower).

Don't:

- Eat stale leftovers.
- Cook with hydrogenated or trans fats.
- Use old or stale oils.
- Buy highly processed foods with a long list of additives.
- Buy boxed and canned foods except for those with the fewest, simplest additives, like citric acid and water.

At the beginning I told you my story about going "all pure," which would have been considered extreme a decade ago. Now more than ever I feel that it's the normal American diet that is extreme. Purity in all of our food and water is a basic demand that everyone should make. If you have the intention of a completely pure diet, a mountain of medical evidence exists to back you up.

You don't need any refined white sugar to satisfy the desire for sweetness—honey, maple syrup, and other natural sweeteners are part of whole foods and therefore much better for you. You don't need alcohol for stimulation, because its toxic effects cannot be ignored. In terms of weight alone, alcohol interferes with insulin levels by giving your body a sudden jolt of the simplest sugar in nature, which is what alcohol basically is. You don't need additives and preservatives when their long-term effect on the body isn't known, and with new ones being added all the time. You don't need flavor enhancers since all they do is dull your natural sensitivity to taste.

Set yourself the goal of a completely pure diet, and then go for it with enthusiasm. Don't change your life out of anxiety. *Purity* is a positive theme that is meant to increase your sense of joyful living.

You can make your diet purer right this minute with a simple step: Get rid of whatever is stale and old. If your nose tells you that something's not fresh, throw it out. The chemistry of going stale is complex, but in the larger picture, do you want *stale* to be a theme in your life? *Fresh*, *pure*, and *natural* are such desirable words that advertisers use them constantly for products that are far from fresh, pure, and natural (for example, the "fresh" taste of artificial whipped cream filled with processed fats, additives, and artificial ingredients).

More and more, preventive medicine has been concentrating on the damaging effects of oxidation, the same process that causes iron to rust, wine to go bad, and a cut apple to turn brown. In the body the process is much more complicated, but major actors are free-floating oxygen atoms, known as *free radicals*, that attach themselves to tissues with damaging effects. Some free radicals come from the environment (in air pollution and cigarette smoke, for example), but they are chiefly produced by the body. The collateral damage of free radical formation is responsible for illness and aging. Many of the most common illnesses of our society are linked to free radical damage, including the following:

Cancer
Heart disease
Stroke
Diabetes
Arthritis
Osteoporosis
Inflammatory bowel disease
Glaucoma
Retinal degeneration
Alzheimer's disease

Other damaging effects are visible in the mirror. Wrinkling skin, graying hair, and stiffening joints are also the result of free radicals. In relation to overweight, if you are eating too much food, and it includes old, stale food and leftovers, you are aggravating the damage. I am not promoting a fear of free radicals, because their action in the body is complicated and not completely understood (for example, free radicals increase dramatically at the site of wounds and cuts, rushing in as part of the healing process).

Fresh foods aren't oxidized, and even better, some foods contain antioxidants that may counter the damaging effects of free radicals. One of the reasons that nuts and naturally processed vegetable oils are beneficial is that they are a prime source of vitamin E, one of the best antioxidants (its benefits are lost, however, if your stored almonds or olive oil have gotten old and stale). All told, there are things you can do that increase free radical production and other things that can limit it. The following factors increase free radical formation:

Smoking
Environmental pollution
Alcohol

Radiation, including excessive sunlight exposure

Barbecued and smoked meats

Aged and fermented foods, including cheeses

Chemotherapy drugs

High intake of saturated and hydrogenated fats (hydrogenated fats, most commonly vegetable shortening, are made solid through chemical processing)

Stress and stress hormones

The body has a system for deactivating free radicals, and there are ways that you can help the process, including the following:

Eat more antioxidant-rich foods—fresh fruits and vegetables, grains, nuts, and beans

Use antioxidant-rich herbs and spices liberally—dill, coriander, rosemary, sage, thyme, mint, fennel, ginger, and garlic

Take antioxidant vitamins—A, C, and E

Eliminate tobacco, excessive alcohol, and nonessential drugs

Reduce your stress

Meditate

Being overweight doesn't tend to move people in the right direction for preventing these disorders. It's well documented that obesity is linked to consuming far too much fat, empty calories in sugar, all kinds of processed food, and meals at fast-food chains. If you make choices that favor *purity*, you will begin to turn this around.

But what about noncompliance, the inability to follow good advice? The answer is to make *purity* part of your plan for fulfillment.

"Pure" fulfillment: Imagine that you are considering what to order for lunch, and your eye lands on "Mexican combination plate with beef enchiladas and refried beans." You're hungry, and your mouth starts to water at the prospect. Eating beef enchiladas would be

satisfying, and if you deny yourself, your brain registers it as deprivation. You need to find a new choice that feels just as fulfilling. In this situation, some people will sigh and say, "I want to be good. Just bring me a salad," which is sensible and nutritious, but it's hard to consider a salad as fulfilling as a fatty enchilada when that's what you're in the mood for.

So here's a new way to think about it, using the theme of *purity*. The enchiladas are made of beef, which was almost certainly raised with hormones to speed muscle production. The cheese is full of saturated fats, and if the meat was seared on a grill over a flame, the smoke from charred drippings is a known carcinogen. These things don't fit the life you want to lead. Now make a small shift to fish tacos. The fish will contain omega-3 oils and be digested much more easily; the cabbage or lettuce on top has vitamin C and antioxidants. You will still be getting a spicy Mexican meal (the hot chilies are good for pulmonary function, clearing the passageways in your lungs), and the calories are much lower. Even if you keep the cheese, fish tacos add to your theme of *purity*. Deciding to order them brings a small victory that adds positively to your whole story.

(Note: Medical science also helps out here. Your blood is composed of blood cells that float in a clear, straw-colored liquid known as plasma. After you eat a plate of beef enchiladas or a cheeseburger, your plasma gets clouded for up to 6 hours afterward—it's quite a startling sight to see the difference when someone's plasma is extracted after they've eaten such a meal. The cloudiness is from molecules of animal fat that remain solid at body temperature. They easily get deposited in the microscopic cracks in the walls of your arteries, building up deposits of plaque like dirty snowflakes filling a crack in the sidewalk.)

Now you have something delicious to eat that won't feel like deprivation, because you've added a new kind of fulfillment—a higher kind—based on your power to write the story you want for yourself.

If you win two or three victories like this every day, your story will be moving in the right direction, and so will your body.

Action Step:
Make It Pure.

The next time you are choosing what to eat, run your choice through a mental filter, using the best information available to you (from labels, the Internet, etc.).

- How fatty is it?
- Is there hidden sugar?
- Are there additives and adulterants?
- Is there good antioxidant potential?
- How fresh are the ingredients?
- How processed are the ingredients?

This kind of rundown becomes quite easy and quick once you're used to it. Now challenge yourself to find the most delicious food that passes your mental quiz.

When you get into the spirit of it, this action step turns into an enjoyable challenge. You know that *you are eating the food that fits the story you want to live*. Don't choose something you don't really want—disappointment and deprivation aren't allowed. The whole point is to add to your fulfillment, not subtract from it. As a bonus to your emotional satisfaction, your body will almost always feel better an hour after you have had pure food than if you ate fatty or processed food.

If you want your life to be pure and free of the opposite theme, *toxicity*, all of these changes will give you a new story and a new body at the same time.

Energy

Energy begins with food
that is nourishing and natural.
The five senses add to the vibrancy
of food, which is an added source of energy.
The highest kind of energy comes
from the joy of eating, which calls
upon your mind and emotions.

Your body needs fuel, so the theme of *energy* begins with extracting calories as food gets digested. But much more is implied in this theme. The food you eat should add to the vibrancy, excitement, and joy in your life—these are the kinds of energy that bring true fulfillment, far beyond blood sugar levels. What you don't want is to promote the opposite theme, *inertia*, which is flat and dull. When you look at food in terms of the bigger theme, here are some guidelines:

Do:

- Eat to feel energized. Eat less when you are inactive.
- Choose the freshest ingredients you can find.
- Stop eating when you are nicely satisfied and go no further.
- Choose lighter, more easily digested food.
- Avoid heavy animal-based fats and refined sugar.
- Make your food colorful and pleasing to the eye.
- Satisfy as many of the senses as possible, including taste, smell, and texture.

Don't:

- Eat until you are stuffed.
- Go for quick-fix energy boosts, such as highly caffeinated en-

ergy drinks and sugar-loaded bars. (Tea and coffee are the best energy boosts, being natural and noncaloric.)

- Make yourself foggy with too much sugar, fat, or alcohol.
- Shovel your food in without enjoying each bite.
- Choose the same foods every day, without variety.
- Neglect the visual aspect of an attractive plate of food.

Energy is a perfect example of how intimately connected mind, body, and emotions are. You can walk away from the table feeling buoyant and joyful, the perfect outcome to feasting. Or with the same calorie intake, you can walk away feeling as if nothing has happened—the meal was just a mechanical routine. For this reason, *energy* is a holistic theme whose aim is not to extract nutrients as efficiently as possible but to make eating a joyful experience.

I remember reading a memoir in which the author, who had fallen in love with a European, found herself on a brisk day in the Alps. It was May, and the scenery was stunning. She had every reason to feel uplifted, and she was. But what stuck in her mind centered on food. The little group of friends she was with were having a picnic that consisted of fresh-baked bread, tiny new peas just picked from the garden, and creamery butter. At that moment, in such a setting, these simple foods became part of a magical memory.

Yet on their own, peas are peas, bread is bread, and butter is butter. The amount of calories they contain is fixed and unchanging, no matter whether you pull them out of your refrigerator, where they've been sitting awhile, or eat them at the peak of freshness. But we are sensitive on other levels, and each one has its own energy signature. There's no scientific measure to tell you why a freshly plucked rose handed to you by someone you love isn't the same as a refrigerated rose packaged in a plastic sheath at the supermarket. There's no way to quantify this, but the energy is certainly different.

When you look at the whole package of *energy*, the food you eat should match the story you want to live, which means:

As **fresh** as possible, without dullness, repetition, and routine.

As **colorful** as possible, giving delight to the eyes. Food is a rainbow brought down to earth.

As **cheerful** as possible, maximizing moments of happiness and pleasure. There's wisdom in the Jewish proverb, "Better to eat straw in a manger than a feast in a house of discord."

It's ironic that many Americans feel they have to go abroad to enjoy eating. They bask in the slow lunches that take hours on a terrace in Tuscany. They feel excited in a Parisian café where pride in cooking and eating can be felt in the air. By contrast, eating at home tends to be quick, efficient, and routine. Fuel gets put into your stomach. Otherwise, there is no nourishment to the senses or the soul. The modernist architect Le Corbusier called a house "a machine for living," which sounds rather bleak. It's just as bleak when meals turn into pit stops for refueling.

Your body isn't looking for fuel the way a diesel truck is. It's looking for a myriad of nutrients. The ones that work as fuel are few and easy to outline:

Carbohydrates convert quickly into energy as measured through blood sugar levels.

Proteins break down into energy more slowly and are largely used to rebuild cells, not for providing energy you can feel.

Fats are directed to be stored in the body and take the longest time to turn into energy.

To a nutritionist, carbohydrates are the body's basic fuel and should form the largest segment of everyone's daily diet. A small amount of protein is needed every 24 hours to rebuild tissues (about 3 to 6 ounces, which is much less than most people assume; one sizable portion of lean fish is adequate). Fats are necessary but can be reduced to as little as 1 to 2 tablespoons a day of added oils without harming your health; in fact, severe fat restriction is the only known way to reverse clogged coronary arteries—your body won't call upon these crannies of hardened fat unless deprived of any other source in your diet.

Into this clear picture all kinds of confusion has been introduced, particularly regarding carbohydrates. Decades ago, athletes who ate at the training table were given red meat, on the assumption that increased protein was necessary to build muscle mass, and with more muscles, an athlete should be able to reach maximum performance. But in a series of experiments performed at Yale University, two groups of athletes were put on exercise bicycles and told to pedal to the point of exhaustion. The athletes who performed best weren't the ones who ate protein but the ones who ate carbohydrates before a game. The practice of "carbing up" was born.

In order to give you quick energy, carbs are processed by insulin produced in the pancreas, a rapid-fire mechanism that takes mere seconds if you drink a soda or any other form of sucrose, the simplest of sugars and the fastest to enter your system. It seems that a lot of problems would be averted if Americans didn't load their bodies with refined, or simple sugar. In nature, carbs are complex. They take longer to break down, which helps even out blood sugar, while refined white sugar causes blood sugar to spike. Just as important, natural carbs are packaged into whole food, so a buffer is created by fats and proteins; taken straight, refined white sugar has no such buffer.

Unfortunately, the implications are worse if you gain weight. Americans have long risked a condition of insulin overload (hyperinsulinemia) that is due to injecting too much quick fuel through refined white sugar and high-fructose corn syrup. Even though the latter is based on fructose, which isn't as simple a sugar as sucrose (fructose occurs naturally in fruits and many vegetables), the refining process in making corn syrup removes this advantage.

What troubles doctors is that there's a seeming epidemic of hyper-insulinemia, and the condition is a vicious circle: the more insulin your body produces, the less effective your body is at extracting energy. Fat gets deposited, and the fat secretes hormones that heighten insulin levels, making it even less effective. Meanwhile, diabetes lurks on the horizon, along with links to high blood pressure and a host of other disorders. You can't necessarily judge through symptoms whether you have hyperinsulinemia, but the telltale signs are similar to those of diabetes:

- Fatigue
- Headaches
- Excessive thirst
- Muscle weakness
- Foggy thinking
- Trembling

Rather than going on a symptom safari, however, it's better to stand back and realize that the vicious circle between overweight and excess insulin needs to be broken. A little vigilance makes all the difference.

Breaking a Vicious Circle

Eat the natural carbs contained in whole foods (fruits, vegetables, cereals).

Don't drink sugary sodas; cut out refined white sugar; and use honey, maple syrup, and other natural sweeteners. Use all sweeteners moderately.

Reduce your intake of hidden sugar in processed foods.

For grains and cereals, prefer whole grains over refined ones.

Eat complete meals with several kinds of foods rather than

snacks—give yourself a buffer between the sugar you eat and your blood sugar.

The good news is that losing weight will take care of excessive insulin in most people. Type 2 diabetes, which is now widespread as a result of the obesity epidemic, generally reverses once people get back to their ideal weight. It's good for everyone, even if your blood sugar is normal, to pay attention to the starches and sugars in common foods. Recently attention has been focused on the glycemic index (GI), which ranks each food according to how complex its carbs are. The numbers indicate how quickly a particular food gets converted to glucose, or blood sugar. Slow is better than fast because it prevents spikes in blood sugar, delivering a more even, consistent flow of energy. (Eating the right foods doesn't solve the problem entirely, however. If you eat too much to begin with, the overload on your digestive tract won't be beneficial. In addition, carrying excess weight, particularly belly fat, causes the fat cells to secrete hormones that confuse and impair the signals for hunger and satiation that are bound up with insulin and glucose—in short, the best strategy is to make good choices about how to eat and to return to your ideal weight.)

Since you are learning a mind-body approach to weight control, I don't think it's helpful to fret over glycemic values any more than it is to fret over calories. It's enough to know that refined and processed foods are on the wrong end of the glycemic index, while whole foods tend to be on the right end. Take a glance online at a published version of the GI, which ranks high-glycemic (bad) and low-glycemic (good) foods. This will be enough to give you the lay of the land.

Moreover, the GI isn't infallible. Glycemic values vary from person to person, they can cover a wide range within a single food, and the effect on blood sugar over time isn't listed. A rough guideline is good enough. There are a few surprises, like potatoes and parsnips, which are high on the glycemic scale even though they are whole foods. White bread and white rice, which also have a high glycemic index, go through a refining process. The key words to avoid are *refined*, *processed*, and *manufactured*, as Dr. Andrew Weil likes to remind us.

The most important thing about the *energy* theme is to look beyond the food-as-fuel issue. Eating gives you energy, but it should also invigorate your life.

Action Step:
Eating for Energy

Before you eat, ask yourself:

- Am I in a good mood?
- Is this meal going to be a positive experience?
- Is the food attractive and appealing?
- Can I devote my full attention to enjoying myself?

If the answer is *yes* to all of these questions, you will be getting the best energy from your food. If the answer is *no*, then don't eat, or postpone eating until the negative elements have changed.

Another tip is to eat to the point where you feel satisfied but not stuffed. Stop eating when there's still space in your stomach. Halfway through a meal, put down your fork, and wait 5 to 10 minutes. Check to see if you're still hungry, and then decide if you need more to eat.

As always, don't deprive yourself; make it satisfying to say, "I am adding energy to my story." Since that is the story you want to live, every choice that boosts the theme of *energy* and opposes the theme of *inertia* is a small victory.

Balance

Maintaining your ideal weight
is a physical sign that you are in balance.
Feeling contented and fulfilled
shows that your mind and emotions
have found balance.

Balance doesn't deserve to sound boring or dull. It should be considered precious, like the golden mean, a perfect state in which everything exists in the right proportion. The opposite theme, *imbalance*, means that something has been pushed to extremes. The more extreme, the harder it is for the mind-body system to return to balance. Our society glories in all kinds of extremes, and risk-taking is promoted as an exciting way to live. The story is different as viewed by your body, which reacts to extreme situations as stress, releasing stress hormones like cortisol that are meant to be temporary and fleeting but can course through the body all day and ultimately contribute to hypertension or osteoporosis. When you are out of balance, including the state of overweight, your body fat triggers a harmful array of stress hormones, leading to hidden imbalances throughout the system. Here I concentrate on the dietary side of *balance*, one of the most valuable themes to bring into your life.

Do:

- Eat when you are in a balanced emotional state.
- Consume a wide variety of fresh foods.
- Attend to basics like drinking enough water and getting enough sleep.
- Eat at regular hours with balanced intervals in between.
- Vary your calorie intake to balance your activity level.

Don't:

- Eat the same few foods every day.
- Go on a "mono diet," where one "magic" food dominates your intake.
- Sit down to eat in a bad mood.
- Eat when you are tired or exhausted.
- Shun one food group all the time, such as whole grains, fresh fruits, or vegetables.
- Let excess fat begin to unbalance your meals.

My training in endocrinology gave me a head start regarding balance, because the study of hormones is all about balance. These naturally produced chemicals of the endocrine system tell the body how to sleep, eat, grow, have sex, and respond to stress. Being overweight is a state of imbalance involving five hormones:

Insulin
Cortisol
Leptin
Ghrelin
Adiponectin

The first two have become widely known, since insulin is key in digestion, blood sugar levels, and energy. Cortisol is recognized as a major stress hormone. But the larger truth is that all five of these hormones interact with one another. Leptin and ghrelin are tied into appetite but also sleep, as is cortisol. Adiponectin, which has the same root as *adipose* or fat, regulates fatty acid breakdown; when you go on a fast, only to find afterward that everything you eat winds up around your waist or on your thighs, the reason is that this hormone promotes fat retention. The body is reacting to what it senses as a famine by storing more fat for the future.

A balance of these five hormones leads to overall balance in body weight. It appears that obesity has two basic types. One is based on excess cortisol due to stress, and the fat is deposited as belly fat. This kind of fat is the worst you can have, because it secretes ghrelin, the so-called hunger hormone. It's a double whammy because the more fat you eat, the hungrier you are, while the fat you put on also makes you hungrier. The other type of obesity is traced back to insulin and the blood sugar problems we've discussed.

Drug companies work constantly to develop new pharmaceuticals that will rebalance hormones. But unless you need drugs for a disease condition like type 1 diabetes, adding more chemicals to the delicate endocrine system isn't the way. Hormones get out of balance when your life is out of balance. Being in balance means:

Good sleep
Reduced stress
Proper food
Positive emotions
Sense of well-being

If you fiddle with hormones, you are putting the cart before the horse. Instead, all you need to do is balance your life; hormonal balance will follow naturally.

The reason that the theme of *balance* may seem boring—and is so often ignored—doesn't come as a surprise. Leading a balanced life sounds like something you settle for after middle age sets in. We glamorize youth, a time when impulses ran free, there were no responsibilities, and excitement was fueled by new adventures (and a surge of hormones). But it's just as true that adolescents have the highest rates of suicide and traffic accidents, that they are afflicted with insecurity and anxiety over the future, and that misbegotten adventures can turn out badly.

I'm not intentionally painting a gloomy picture for its own sake.

Most people eat today the way they ate in childhood and adolescence. Think of the following labels that fit our social concept of being a teenager:

Breaking the rules
Running wild
Going crazy
Rebelling against authority
Bingeing

If you transfer these labels to how you eat, bad things will happen. I'm not being judgmental. As far as your body is concerned, you aren't breaking the rules or acting like a rebel when you consume six beers, a plate of chili fries, and half a pint of Chunky Monkey. You are, however, throwing your body into drastic imbalance. As you burden your digestive tract, your body is forced to shut down or minimize other functions that need energy and attention. It can't send fire trucks to every fire; the worst one has to be dealt with first.

The chronic imbalance of overweight, if it continues long enough, leads to the following:

Dullness and tiredness
Poor sleep
Uncontrolled appetite
Decreased sex drive
Incipient health problems (a wide range beginning with joint pain, high blood pressure, type 2 diabetes, coronary artery disease, etc.)

Theoretically, almost all of these effects could be cured with a ten-second lecture to yourself that begins, "Grow up. Act more mature. Take responsibility." But that would be futile. Maturity, and the balance it brings, aren't compulsory. If you harbor beliefs that cling to adolescence, you won't elect to lead a more balanced life—why not keep fantasizing about a glamorous one where youth never ends?

As with all the themes in this book, *balance* has to be more appealing than the alternatives. Of course, one appeal comes from knowledge and experience. If you remember what it felt like to be wasted after a night of bingeing, your desire to repeat it won't be strong. But I'm not at all confident that negative motivation works. The brain's first-response team consists of drives, impulses, appetites, and desires. This team doesn't listen to "You'll be sorry later." It knows no later, only now. (Adding morality doesn't help, either, or we'd all have a needlepoint cushion with the old Protestant proverb, "Sin in haste, repent at leisure.")

Action Step:
Balance Feels Good—Try It.

The positive spin on negative motivation is this: *Do the right thing, then see how good it feels.* You can put this into practice today. Try any of the activities listed on page 78, then half an hour later, check in with yourself. Notice how good you feel. Mentally register any positive sensations that you notice, naming them to yourself:

I feel focused.
I'm alert.
I'm thinking clearly, without drowsiness.
I'm ready for action; I have energy.
I feel satisfied.
I feel content.

Here are the suggested activities, which you can test one at a time or combine however you like:

1. Eat a light, satisfying meal.

2. As already mentioned, leave a little empty space in your stomach rather than filling up.

3. Drink a nonalcoholic beverage.

4. Skip dessert.

5. If you are in pleasant company, cut your food intake by half.

6. Have a small serving of protein accompanied by colorful, tasty vegetables in abundance.

7. Eat a vegetarian meal where you like all the foods.

Notice that you aren't imposing "balance" as a tiresome commonplace but putting into action a new way of eating. The theme of *balance* is mature because it is measured by how you feel afterward. Craving immediate stimulation isn't bad; after all, the delicious taste of food is experienced here and now. The mark of maturity is to balance *immediate* and *long-term*. If a benefit is too long term, it won't work. But a delay of half an hour does work, because how you feel is still connected to the meal you just enjoyed.

Balance is a natural state, but so is imbalance, which adds another piece to the puzzle. Your body is a miracle of adaptability. It can adapt to the elevation in Death Valley, the lowest place on earth, or to the high Andes of Peru, more than 16,000 feet above sea level. We are omnivores; our bodies can adapt to almost any diet, as opposed to a panda, who will die without tender green bamboo shoots, or a koala, who cannot survive without eucalyptus leaves (and a huge amount of them, since the koala and panda have never evolved a completely efficient digestive system to go with their diets—both animals must eat constantly during their waking hours, and even then they derive so little energy that the rest of the time is spent sleeping).

The mechanism that lies behind adaptation is known as *homeostasis*, a special kind of balance. If you stir a spoonful of sugar into your morning coffee, the sugar will dissolve evenly throughout, and so any sip of coffee, whether from the bottom or the top of the cup, will have the same balance of sugar and liquid. Your body couldn't survive in such a static, even state. Thousands of chemicals require their own unique balance, which is always shifting. The bloodstream is a superhighway carrying every imaginable kind of message to and from the brain. Your muscles and heart must respond to your demand for action at a moment's notice, causing changes in blood flow, heart rate, and oxygen consumption automatically.

Homeostasis is like a rubber band that can snap back into place after it is stretched out of shape. Going out of balance is highly beneficial, if what we're talking about is exercising instead of sitting still, pushing the limits of your creativity instead of following the same routine, being proactive instead of resigned and passive. As it applies to eating, homeostasis is incredibly adaptive to all kinds of consumption, from gorging to extreme fasting. But just as you can put demands on your muscles to move, the automatic process of digestion allows for all kinds of interventions:

You can skip a meal or not eat altogether.

You can put food in your mouth to compensate for negative feelings.

You can eat to your heart's content, regardless of how much.

You can eat to forget your troubles.

We've already been discussing these things, but the point here is that the messages you insert into the process either work to balance the mind-body system or throw it into imbalance—and your body must adapt, without choice or complaint. Cells have a life of their own—a complex, fascinating life—but when the mind calls, they must listen.

The Most Negative Messages

Depression
Lack of sleep
Bad body image
Low self-esteem
Failure
Loss
Grief

If you were Sherlock Holmes looking for a villain in hiding, Mister X would turn out to be one of these things, silently throwing your body into a state of stress, chaos, chemical imbalance, and so on. Lacking a Sherlock Holmes, the only sleuth is your awareness.

Here is where *balance* becomes a positive. Taking a balanced attitude to negative messaging brings healing. Instead of rejecting the message or forcing yourself into positive thinking that is just a coat of paint, you can intervene in the name of balance.

Healing Interventions

Be easy with yourself.
Take extra time when making choices.
Exercise patience if you backslide.
Offer yourself reassurance.
Seek comfort from warm friends.
Give yourself peace and solace.
Minimize stressful experiences.

All of these things apply to losing weight, because carrying excess weight is an imbalanced state for the mind-body system, just as much as losing your job or grieving over a loved one you've lost. Your body doesn't have words to label what is happening to it, but if it did, its message would always be, "I'm doing the best I can to get us back into balance."

Understand this message without words, and then intervene by giving your body what it needs to rebalance itself. If you consider the healing interventions listed earlier, their opposite hinders the return to balance:

What Hurts Healing?

Being hard on yourself
Demanding instant solutions
Seeing yourself as a failure
Repressing how you really feel
Being impatient and thoughtless
Stabbing at answers without thinking them through
Self-judgment

I said at the outset that you don't have to psychoanalyze yourself to lose weight with a mind-body approach. That's still true. But you do have to be aware. The most basic awareness applies to balance—either you are balanced or you aren't. Since an overweight body by definition is out of balance, it's up to you to help it return to balance with healing thoughts and deeds.

Knowing that you are healing yourself is one of the biggest satisfactions that the theme of *balance* brings.

Making It Personal:
Purify Effortlessly.

Although its first aim is to purify by removing toxins, doing a mild detox once a week benefits the other two themes at the same time. Your body gets to rebalance itself without the normal call for energy that is necessary for the digestive process. Traditional medicine in every culture has recommended some kind of purification ritual, and the wisdom behind this is holistic: when I take one day a week to follow a mild purification regimen, I feel lighter in every way, including my mood and my thoughts.

The basics of purification all come from natural products. In your general diet it's good to include foods with purifying properties, including the following:

Kale, cabbage, and broccoli

Oranges, lemons, and grapefruit

Mung beans

Watercress

Artichokes

Asparagus

Beets

Ginger

Garlic

Apples

Sesame seeds

Almonds

For a day set aside to purify the system, three groups of food are time-tested; they figure into my weekly routine now, without fail.

Oils: Various oils have a laxative effect but are also considered to have detox properties. On my purification day I take a mixture of four oils—olive, sesame, flaxseed, and evening primrose—easily found in health food stores already made up. I use 1 or 2 table-spoons of the mixture in the morning, taken by itself or with food.

Fiber: The medical benefits of fiber are well documented, es-pecially as a buffer in the intestine—moderating cholesterol, for example, and possibly protecting the wall of the intestine from carcinogens. The natural fiber in vegetables is easier on your body than bran and other grain-based fiber (these can have an abrasive effect on the intestinal wall). I take 2 tablespoons of powdered fiber in the morning, mixed with club soda. Some delicious varieties of this fiber are sold in health food stores.

Juices: Juice fasts have been popular for decades, but they have been criticized for relying so heavily on sugar, and in any event they shouldn't last more than a few days. On my purification day I have only vegetable juice, followed in the evening by a broth-based vegetable soup like minestrone. The juice extracted from leafy green vegetables is especially high in phytonutrients (more about these later), which are micronutrients known to have antioxidant properties. Herbal and wheatgrass juices are even more packed with concentrated micronutrients. If possible, fresh-squeezing your own or buying them fresh-squeezed is best.

Vegetable juices, except for tomato juice (technically a fruit), supply almost no calories, so be cautious about jolting your system by suddenly removing all caloric intake. I have done purification for more than one day several times and find it easy to sustain, but for anyone the key is that you feel fulfilled—no deprivation.

Fruit juices have fallen out of favor, in part because separating the juice from a fruit's fiber (the pulp in an orange, the peel of an apple) reduces it to being a surge of sugar. Because they contain fructose, fresh fruit juices supply energy without putting any pressure on the digestive tract. But they must be taken in moderation, since you don't want to throw your insulin levels off with jolts of sugar on an empty stomach. Mixing the juice with fiber in the morning works well. For the rest of the day, sip juice diluted with warm water, always in moderation.

My weekly purification, based on oils, fiber, and juices, feels like the best day of the week. I have the satisfaction of devoting quality attention to my body and listening to what it has to say. The messages of lightness and energy are rewarding, so there's no sense of deprivation.

If you want to go further—as we all know, purification programs exist all around us, as close as a Google search—start out with the effortless steps just outlined, then see if other purification steps work well for you. Tune in to your body. Suffering isn't purification; being hard on your body isn't being cruel to be kind—it's just cruel.

The tradition of purification has given us some time-honored recommendations:

- Make your purification day a day of rest. Devoting time to meditation is even better.
- Going into silence for a day adds the element of self-reflection and calmness.
- Fasting can be tried in all of its guises. A moderate fast for an adult male would be 1,000 to 1,500 calories; for an adult female, 700 to 1,100 calories. Fasting also includes doing without meat and alcohol and drinking plenty of water during the day. It's also good to monitor your energy level, taking a small amount of food if you feel dull or listless. (More serious discomfort means that you should stop fasting immediately.)
- Cleansing for purification appeals to many people consulting a wide span of healers. At the Chopra Center we use specialized herbs and fruit extracts combined with *panchakarma*, the five purification methods of Ayurveda. Panchakarma is done under

clinic conditions with trained professionals. But for many people, "doing a cleanse" generally means taking a single purifying food all day or for several days (like the green vegetable soup known as Bieler broth) or dosing with a mixture of olive oil and lemon juice. If you're in good health, a cleansing, although rigorous, can add to your sense of healthy well-being. See how your body reacts and pay attention to its messages.

"What Should I Eat?"

Power Points

- The principles of Ayurveda, India's traditional "science of life," provide a reliable guide for modern eating.
- Ayurveda treats food as part of your whole life experience.
- There are six tastes in Ayurveda, each with a different effect on mind and body.
- Once you know the six tastes, they can be expanded to emotions and other areas of life.
- Ayurveda respects the wisdom of the body, looking for signs of imbalance long before disease symptoms appear.

From the outset I've wanted to show how a weight-loss book isn't the same as a diet book. Crash diets have always been ineffective, and many aren't good for the body. But *diet* has another meaning: an overall way of eating. Human beings are omnivores. We have the ability to digest almost any nutrient found in nature. This great gift is also a drawback, however, because finding the best diet leads in so many directions. What should you eat today and tomorrow and for years to come? It's a natural question, and there's an answer. But it's not really contained in a list of groceries.

Once I started eating better myself, I arrived at a philosophy of food that I believe in completely: The best diet should do the following at every meal:

Keep me healthy
Not contribute to the aging process
Give me a sense of lightness and energy
Refresh my senses
Send the right messages to my body
Increase my sense of well-being

You know the importance of several of these points already. To deliver the whole package, the Chopra Center promotes well-being for a lifetime. At the cutting edge of medicine is the realization that dietary choices can prevent disease and aging. For example, the Centers for Disease Control in 2012 announced that up to two-thirds of cancers may be preventable. Half of these cancers are related to obesity, it is now thought. Another large segment is related to smoking and other environmental toxins.

There is no magic bullet in the area of diet and cancer. It cannot be said that food A prevents cancer, for two reasons: The interaction of food with the body is incredibly complex, and the causes of cancer are just as complex—there are many kinds of cancer. Their causes involve multiple factors, and only a few can be ascribed to a single cause. If you don't know a precise cause, you can't name what blocks the cause. We are left with a promising picture anyway: of a natural diet rid of toxins; foods eaten in whole form rather than being processed; and the elimination of excess fat, sugar, and salt because of their known links to a whole range of lifestyle disorders. Heart disease has long been considered a lifestyle disorder, meaning that positive lifestyle change greatly reduces your risk of contracting this disease. Now it appears that cancer will join the list. In other words, each of us can become more self-reliant in remaining healthy for a lifetime, with minimal dependence on doctors, drugs, and surgery. This isn't just good medical advice—it will turn out in the end to be the best prevention regimen in existence.

Let me outline in detail how my philosophy of food works.

The Ayurvedic Way

The principles I follow at every meal are aligned with the time-honored system of Ayurveda in India, which translates from Sanskrit as "science of life." I have purposely avoided using Ayurvedic terminology in this book, since many people are unfamiliar with the Indian tradition or find it esoteric and somewhat difficult to conceptualize. But since the program at the Chopra Center is based on Ayurveda, let me put Ayurveda into everyday terms for anyone asking, "What should I eat?"

To begin with, Ayurveda is about personal experience. Eating isn't isolated on its own. A harmonious meal fits into a harmonious day. When you eat a delicious dish, you don't consciously experience the 323 calories, 25 grams of protein, 7 grams of fat, and 40 grams of carbohydrates it contains. Instead, you vividly experience your five senses and the feelings that eating evokes. You hear soup bubbling on the stove and experience comfort. You feel the creamy texture of a spoonful of custard and have a moment of delight. In Ayurveda, harmony is all-embracing. It includes the vibrancy of colorful foods and the pleasure of a well-set table. Every sensation carries its own message; every message is received by your cells.

In keeping with this Ayurvedic understanding, we pay more attention at the Chopra Center to the personal experience of eating than to measuring each specific quantity of nutrition. Science has done its work in breaking down the healthful ingredients in food. But knowledge has to be turned into experience and then into applied wisdom. The nutritional label on a bag of potato chips supplies knowledge. Choosing not to buy the potato chips gives you the chance to experience something better. Applied wisdom runs deeper. Consider the following Bible verse:

Better a dry crust with peace and quiet than feasting in a house of strife. (Proverbs 17:1)

One finds applied wisdom there. I think more of the same can be found in Ayurveda, for anyone who is open to its brand of wisdom.

One piece of applied wisdom is "First, do no harm," the same instruction given to physicians in the Hippocratic oath. The food you take in shouldn't interfere with the body's natural state of well-being. Second, eat food that comes as close as possible to being harvested that day. Your palate can immediately tell the difference, and according to Ayurveda, so can the rest of your body, because taste is the principal way that we instinctively shape our diet.

At the Chopra Center we recommend that you eliminate or minimize the use of *FLUNC* foods, an acronym for food that is:

Frozen
Leftover
Unnatural
Nuked (microwaved)
Canned

In Ayurveda, the fresher the food, the more life force, or *prana*, is available. This principle applies to all categories of food, including not only fruits and vegetables but also meat (including fish), eggs, dairy, and grain. While we encourage you to move toward a plant-based diet, we believe that high-quality (and organic where possible) meat (including chicken and fish) and dairy, in moderation, can be enjoyed as part of a balanced diet.

More Tips for Maximum Freshness

Choose fruits and vegetables that are locally grown, freshly harvested, and prepared as soon as possible after picking. They are more flavorful and delectable, and they send your body the message that it's receiving the highest-quality nutrients. Foods that are stored and shipped great distances are more likely to be affected by oxidation. As soon as a piece of fruit or a vegetable is picked, the process of decomposition begins. A banana turns brown after sitting for an hour because free radical molecules deplete it of its natural antioxidants.

Eat in Season

It's best to eat fruits and vegetables that are in season where you live because they will have the best flavor and nutritional value. If you live in an area where produce isn't available year-round, look for fruits and vegetables that radiate the most life force. If they look and smell fresh, they are most likely to taste good and contain optimal levels of energy and information.

Visit Your Local Farmers Market

Farmers markets not only offer fresh, organic foods that are in season, they are also interesting places to visit, whether on your own or with friends and family. You can learn a lot about food and its benefits by talking with the farmers who grow it—and you'll also be supporting your local economy.

Grow Your Own

Growing your own fruits, vegetables, and herbs can be fun and satisfying. Even if you live in a small apartment, you can try a container garden on a windowsill or balcony. There are many excellent books on organic gardening—choose one that suits your area and climate.

What Does "Natural" Mean?

The terms *natural* and *unnatural* require a little explanation—many labels tout a food product as "natural," a claim that can mean anything the seller wants it to. The U.S. Department of Agriculture (USDA) doesn't strictly define or regulate the use of the word in food labeling except in the category of meat. When you buy a tub of "all-natural" yogurt, it may legally contain toxic pesticides, genetically modified organisms (GMOs), antibiotics, and growth hormones. On the other hand, the legal standards for foods labeled "organic" in the United States are under federal regulations (although there are perennial complaints that inspections tend to be haphazard and loose). In general, choosing fresh organic foods will ensure that you are getting products with the highest levels of purity and vitality.

Natural vs. Organic

	Natural	Organic
Toxic persistent pesticides and herbicides	Allowed	Not allowed
GMOs	Allowed	Not allowed
Antibiotics	Allowed	Not allowed
Growth hormones	Allowed	Not allowed
Irradiation	Allowed	Not allowed
Animal-welfare regulations	No	Yes
Lower levels of environmental pollution	Not necessarily	Yes
Audit trail from farm to table	No	Yes

Natural vs. Organic (cont.)

	Natural	Organic
Certification required, including regular inspections	No	Yes
Cows required to be on pasture for pasture season	No	Yes
Legal restrictions on materials allowed	No	Yes

Chart adapted from www.stonyfield.com/why-organic/organic-vs-natural

The following chart handily summarizes what we've just discussed.

Eliminate	Favor
Frozen foods	Recently harvested foods, whenever possible
Leftover foods	Freshly prepared foods
Artificial colorings, flavorings, and additives	All-natural ingredients
Microwaved foods	Conventionally prepared foods
Canned foods	Fresh foods, when possible
Refined and processed foods	Fresh organic fruits, vegetables, and dairy products
Genetically modified organisms (GMOs)	Food that hasn't been genetically modified

Mindful-Eating Meditation

To receive the full benefits from the food you eat, your mind must come into play. Hasty, thoughtless eating is unsatisfying, while putting your attention on every bite—mindful eating—is the way to gain real satisfaction. Chewing a single bite of food with total focus is miles away from gulping it down. Some people are amazed at what they've been missing.

The following meditation uses the power of attention to improve digestion and metabolism along with the whole sensory experience.

It should be done when you are eating alone and undistracted. The technique involves slowing down and deliberately intending every movement.

1. Begin by looking at your food and taking it in visually.
2. Become aware of the food's aroma; savor it for a moment.
3. When you taste each bite, intend to taste it fully, without distractions. See which tastes you can identify, using the six Ayurvedic tastes (discussed on pages 94–107) as your guide. Appreciate the texture of each bite as you chew.

This exercise in mindful eating sharpens your awareness; it's not meant as a continual practice. By eating even just one or two meals a week this way, you can gradually transform your relationship with food, achieving a new level of complete nutrition.

A Word About Inflammation

Recent medical research has focused on inflammation as a major contributor to many kinds of disorders, including type 2 diabetes, heart disease, and various cancers. It has long been realized that inflammation is hard to understand, because it is at once a completely necessary process and yet a damaging one. Acute inflammation is the body's natural response to an injury or attack by bacteria, viruses, or fungi. When you sprain your ankle and quickly start to experience heat, swelling, redness, and pain, this is your immune system rushing in to protect and heal the injured tissues. Acute inflammation is temporary, lasting only a few days or weeks at most. Without it, wounds and infections couldn't heal. But fever is a damaging form of acute inflammation, as is the severe inflammation that puts burn victims into shock and threatens their lives.

Not all inflammation is acute: Chronic inflammation is long-term, and can last for several months or even years. Instead of helping the body heal, it stresses cells and tissues, and is linked to chronic illness. There are few symptoms at first to indicate that damage is being done, or even none. Normally, when you are feeling healthy and well, there is no need for the inflammation response, and yet it seems to be present in many people. The cause for this chronic condition is complex and not fully understood, but whenever your body goes out of balance, tissues can become inflamed, with the most likely cause being chronic low-level stress. Excess weight, belly fat, and lack of sleep may be contributors, too, since all are connected with stress hormones and metabolic imbalances. Toxins in herbicides, pesticides, and various chemical additives are suspect, leading some researchers to blame highly refined, processed foods as promoters of inflammation in the body, especially given the widespread use of hormones in animal feed to speed up muscle growth and increase milk production in dairy cows.

Chronic inflammation is also what medical researchers and nutritionists are referring to when they talk about inflammatory foods or diets. Some foods apparently contribute to chronic inflammation, while others help decrease it. Trans fats, sodium, and preservatives are potentially major sources of chronic inflammation. Whole, fresh foods decrease inflammation and provide valuable fiber, which may act as a buffer against inflammation.

In general, if you avoid FLUNC foods and favor fresh, real food, you can be assured that you are offering your body anti-inflammatory nutrition.

The Six Tastes at Every Meal

According to Ayurveda, a simple way to make sure that you are getting a balanced diet is to include every taste in each meal. Six tastes are recognized: the four usual ones—sweet, sour, salty, and bitter— along with two more, pungent and astringent, as described shortly.

Essentially, these six tastes are supplied by the whole range of foods in nature. In the centuries that preceded modern nutrition, including all six in every meal ensured that the major food groups and nutrients were represented, but it also provided a feeling of complete satisfaction, which in Ayurveda is just as important. When you finish a meal feeling satisfied, you will be much less likely to find yourself raiding the refrigerator two hours later, driven by a sense of lack.

The typical American diet tends to be dominated by the three tastes that the makers of snacks and fast food rely on as the most addictive: sweet, sour, and salty (the main flavors of the "special sauce" in a Big Mac, for example). You do need these tastes, Ayurveda says, but in excess they create cravings and therefore lead to imbalance; at the very least, fixating on sweet, sour, and salty is the same as excluding green leafy vegetables, the chief source of bitter taste, and most beans and legumes, which are astringent in the Ayurvedic system. In the Western scheme, these two tastes also act as anti-inflammatories.

To translate Ayurveda into Western terms, the six tastes are the codes that inform your nervous system about a meal's nutritional content. Evolution has matched taste with the benefits of food—this is the wisdom of thousands of years of experience. The experience of taste is so subtle that unlike mammals whose nutritional requirements are satisfied with a narrow range of foods (e.g., lions subsisting on gazelles and other antelopes) or even a single food (e.g., koalas eating only eucalyptus leaves), human beings find too much of a single taste cloying—we range across the entire field of tastes in order to feel satisfied.

Let's look at each taste in detail. Not every source of the six tastes exactly coincides with our usual perception, although most do. I will also mention some potential health benefits, but this requires a caveat. Intensive research is ongoing about how effective certain foods may be in preventing a host of lifestyle disorders, such as heart disease, diabetes, and cancer. Yet the fact that medical research has isolated a promising compound shouldn't be considered proof positive that you will receive a major benefit, nor are Ayurveda's traditional claims a substitute for carefully controlled studies. The important thing is the holistic effect of eating a natural diet in which all the beneficial components of food come into play. Modern medicine is converging with Ayurveda to recognize that chronic disorders have many causes wrapped up with one another; therefore, finding holistic solutions is gaining increased respect after decades of hoping for magic bullets.

Sweet

Sources: Grains, cereals, bread, pasta, nuts, milk, dairy, and oils are all classified as sweet foods, along with all fish, fowl, and other meat products. Besides ripe fruit, there are sweet vegetables, including tomatoes (technically a fruit), sweet peas, corn, yams, and sweet potatoes.

Foods that provide the sweet taste are considered the most nutritious in Ayurveda, rich in carbohydrates, proteins, and fats. Starchy foods that have no added sugar still belong to the sweet category because the action of saliva converts them into sugar. (Refined, processed sugar and corn syrup were unknown in India when Ayurveda was formulated.) If you examine your grocery cart at the checkout counter, you will probably recognize that you consume a greater volume of foods in this category of flavors than any other. The fact that there is added sugar in processed and snack foods boosts the sweet taste beyond healthy limits, as confirmed by nutritionists. Since the sweet category covers a wide range of edible substances from candy to quinoa, it's important to note that at the Chopra Center, we're never referring to refined sugar as a source for the sweet taste. Every taste should be balancing and nutritious; empty calories are far from that. In general, we recommend the following:

- Favor foods that are rich in complex carbohydrates, including at least five daily servings of vegetables. A half cup of most cooked vegetables or a cup of most greens constitutes one vegetable serving. Choose from a wide variety of green and yellow vegetables.

- Reduce your consumption of all foods made with flour. The action of yeast in raised breads turns starch into sugar. Be aware that even if a loaf of bread is labeled "whole wheat" or "whole grain," it is still usually made from grains that have been pulverized into flour rather than from whole or cracked grains. Thus, most whole-wheat bread ranks just as high as its white-bread counterparts on the glycemic index (that is, its carbs are no longer complex but simple, leading to a spike in insulin and blood sugar). Instead of eating bread, focus on eating grains in their natural state, including quinoa, wild and brown rice, millet, and wheat berries. Several delicious recipes for some of these grains appear at the end of the book.

- When you want to have something really sweet, make the sugars as complex as possible, meaning desserts made with whole fruits or eating fruit out of hand. Canned fruits in syrup, as well as fruit juices, are not recommended—their sugars either are simple or have been separated from the peels and other fiber. Don't exceed two or three servings of fruit a day. One apple, peach, pear, or banana; a half cup of cherries; and half a small cantaloupe are examples of one fruit serving.

- Instead of meat and poultry, favor more vegetable sources of protein, including beans, legumes, seeds, and nuts. Although nuts are high in fat, most of it is polyunsaturated or mono-unsaturated fat, which is better for you than the saturated fats found in animal products. Exclude hydrogenated or trans fats, which are created through a chemical process that transforms liquid oils into solid fats. Nuts contain many beneficial phyto-nutrients (which we will discuss in more detail later) and have been shown to lower cholesterol levels.

- Favor fresh, organic dairy products. While there is ongoing controversy about the health benefits of dairy products, our position at the Chopra Center is that as long as you don't have allergies, consuming organic, low-fat dairy products in moderation has a balancing effect and enhances the experience of the six tastes.

- If you are not vegetarian, minimize your intake of red meat, favoring cold-water fish and lean poultry. Keep in mind the eye-opening findings from 2013 about the benefits of a Mediterranean diet for reducing heart disease and strokes. This widely publicized study, conducted in Spain, doesn't claim that a Mediterranean diet reverses heart disease, but rather that it markedly decreased the incidence of heart attacks and strokes compared to the control group, who were told simply to reduce their calories. A Mediterranean diet is high in fish, nuts, fresh fruits and vegetables, and olive oil, with a corresponding decrease in butter, cheese, and red meat compared with the average American diet.

- Favor fats and oils derived from vegetable and fish sources. Your cooking oils should be either monounsaturated, such as olive oil, or polyunsaturated, such as canola, safflower, or sunflower. A small amount of butter (less than 1 tablespoon per day) adds sweet flavor with an acceptable dose of cholesterol.

Help for a Serious Sweet Tooth

Of all the tastes, sweet is the one people most frequently crave. This may be because sweetness has the most settling effect, going back to nursing at the breast. If you crave sweets, make sure that your diet is thoroughly balanced and that you include all six tastes prepared in a delicious way. Completeness is satisfying on its own, far more than a fix of sugar.

If you're eating the six tastes every day and still have sugar cravings, recognize that the desire for a splurge arises from conditioning, much of it social and almost all from childhood. Be easy with yourself as you change any long-term habit. Don't be fanatical about never eating refined sugar—cutting back from the hundred-plus pounds of white sugar in the average American diet is a major accomplishment without reaching total abstinence. As you've probably experienced, whenever you repress a desire and go to extremes to be "pure," there is an inevitable backlash.

One food that can help stop sugar cravings is milk. Milk contains the sweet taste and has a settling effect on the entire physiology in adults, not just infants. If you constantly hanker for sweets and are not vegan, try drinking a cup of warm milk, perhaps as part of your breakfast. You can also use honey to reduce cravings for sweets. Try drinking a cup of warm water with a teaspoon of honey and a squirt of lemon.

Tips for Sugar Cravings

If you find yourself with a major craving for sugar, there are specific tactics you can try.

- Don't eat sugary snacks, like sodas, doughnuts, or candy bars on their own. A jolt of sugar makes your craving worse; it also has the most drastic effect on insulin and blood sugar spikes. Wait until lunch or dinner, when other food groups can buffer the effects of the sugar.
- Try weaning yourself off sugar. For a snack, slice up an apple or other fruit and sprinkle a teaspoon of sugar or honey on top. You will get an intense sugary taste, but the actual amount of sugar ingested will be minimal, and the whole fruit will help buffer it.
- Don't use artificial sweeteners. You may think you are fooling your body with a diet soda, but just the taste is enough to alter your blood sugar and stoke the craving for more sugar.

- Wait 10 minutes before ordering dessert in a restaurant. Have a cup of coffee or tea, or distract yourself with good conversation. Giving your body a chance to register that it isn't hungry goes a long way toward making sugar cravings subside.
- Before you give yourself a fix of sugar, stop, close your eyes, and wait a moment. Ask if you really want to make this choice. If not, the craving will often pass naturally. Even if you give yourself a fix, keep repeating this exercise. The more you give yourself a chance to make the right choice, the higher your rate of success.

If you eat moderately, with awareness, you won't find yourself inhaling a box of cookies despite your best intentions. A few dessert recipes are included at the end of the book, and if you restrict dessert to one or two times a week, your body will easily bounce back into its state of balance. In any event, make the sweet taste a source of pleasure, without attaching the word *guilty*.

Sour

Sources: Foods ranging from feta cheese to vinegar carry the sour taste; the best sources are fresh fruits, including apples, apricots, strawberries, blueberries, raspberries, cherries, grapefruit, grapes, lemons, oranges, pineapples, and tomatoes. Organic yogurt is a good source of the sour taste and provides acidophilus bacteria, which are helpful in balancing the digestive tract.

The sour taste results from the chemical action of organic acids on your taste buds. All acids are perceived as sour, including citric acid, ascorbic acid (vitamin C), and acetic acid (vinegar). A small dose of sour awakens your appetite and enhances your digestion. It may also slow the emptying of your stomach, reducing the insulin-stimulating effect of carbohydrates.

Ayurveda considers fermentation to have unhealthy effects in the body, so getting the sour taste from vinegar and aged cheese isn't recommended. It's already advisable to limit your consumption of aged cheeses because they are usually high in cholesterol and calories. Fresh cheeses like farmer and cottage cheese are more acceptable, although commercial types may involve chemicals to separate the curds and whey. The homemade process uses lemon juice or a small amount of vinegar.

Sour-tasting fruits are associated with some potentially powerful health benefits. They are usually excellent sources of vitamin C and flavonoids, which may protect against heart disease and cancer, according to some studies. They provide soluble fiber, which may reduce the chances of both coronary heart disease and diabetes. Many fermented condiments, such as pickles, green olives, and chutneys, also carry the sour taste. Although they are helpful in stimulating digestion, they are best taken in small amounts. Get the bulk of your servings of sour through abundant helpings of tart fruits, with less from salad dressings and pickled or fermented foods.

Salty

Sources: In addition to common table salt, the salty taste is contained in fish, soy sauce, tamari, seaweed, and cured meats like bacon, sausage, and ham.

Like the taste of sweet, the taste of salt is necessary in moderation and risky when taken to extremes. Salt is the taste of ion-producing minerals on the tongue. These mineral salts, which reflect our heritage from the sea billions of years ago, are essential for your body's chemical balance—in essence, you are a self-enclosed, walking ocean—but a century ago Americans ate less than a third of the salt we typically consume today. Processed and preserved food items usually have high sodium content. Along with canned foods, fast food,

cheese, and condiments, these are the main sources of dietary sodium for Americans.

In Ayurveda, the salty taste promotes digestion, is mildly laxative,
and has a mildly relaxing effect. Too much salt can contribute to fluid
retention and may play a minor role in the development of osteoporosis. Medically, the worry over salt is connected chiefly to high blood
pressure, but there is no easy test to determine whether you are salt
sensitive. Your kidneys are responsible for removing excessive salt
from the body, and they are generally reliable. But as you grow older,
or if your kidneys decline in function for some other reason, salt becomes more risky. The actual amount of salt that your body needs
per day is small, around 0.5 grams, or less than ½ teaspoon. You
can use table salt lightly to suit your taste, but for almost everyone
there's no risk of too little salt in the diet. The most prudent course is
to keep reducing your salt intake steadily until you reach a comfortable minimum. If you reduce your salt gradually, you'll be surprised
at how easily your taste buds will adapt to even the faint taste of salt.

Bitter

Sources: Green and yellow vegetables are the primary sources of the
bitter taste, including bitter greens in salads (chicory, radicchio, arugula, endive), with less-pronounced bitterness in bell peppers, broccoli, celery, chard, eggplant, spinach, and zucchini. Various herbs
also carry the bitter taste and are useful components of a balanced
meal. Chamomile, cilantro, coriander, cumin, dill, fenugreek, licorice, rhubarb, rosemary, saffron, sage, tarragon, and turmeric are
examples of culinary herbs and spices that contain the bitter flavor.

The bitter taste suppresses appetite and has a cooling effect. Combined with sweetness, as in tonic water, it cools the body in the heat
of the day. It balances the cloying effect of too much sweetness and
the tendency of salty foods to make us overeat. Small amounts of the
bitter taste enhance the other flavors of a meal. Also, bitterness can

be used strategically. If you eat bitter greens in a salad at the end of a meal, your appetite will decrease and with it a craving for dessert.

Bitterness reflects the many natural phytochemicals (*phyto* is Latin for "plant") contained in vegetables that in Ayurveda are considered to have age-reversing effects besides being generally healthy. For example, broccoli and cauliflower are rich in phytochemicals known as *isothiocyanates,* which are thought to play a part in preventing cancer and heart disease. Asparagus, green peppers, and cabbage are rich in other flavonoids that may protect against genetic injury, fight infection, and even reduce your risk of memory loss. Beyond diet, most medicinal herbs such as aloe, black cohosh, echinacea, gentian, goldenseal, licorice, passionflower, skullcap, and St. John's wort are predominantly bitter due to their high concentrations of phytochemicals.

Pungent

Sources: Pungency is the spicy taste found in various herbs and spices, along with hot peppers, onions, garlic, ginger, radishes, mustard, and horseradish. It is also found in pungent herbs not thought of as spicy, such as peppermint, basil, thyme, and rosemary.

Pungency, which registers on the tongue as hot or spicy, usually comes from essential oils that are natural antioxidants. In fact, their ability to neutralize decay-causing free radicals may explain why spices were commonly used to preserve food before the invention of refrigeration. The natural chemicals in hot spices are also considered antibacterial in Ayurveda.

Some research studies indicate that the natural compounds contained in the onion family, including leeks, chives, and garlic, may help lower cholesterol levels and blood pressure. Other studies have found that these pungent foods can protect you from carcinogens in the environment. And by opening passageways in the lungs, chilies are sometimes recommended for respiratory conditions and clearing the sinuses. Leaving aside any potential health benefits, in Ayurveda the main attraction of herbs and spices is that they make eating a more varied and colorful experience. Pungency is the most stimulating of the six tastes. Tropical cuisines around the world depend heavily on them to brighten and energize people, counteracting the lethargic effect of a prolonged hot day.

Astringent

Sources: The dry, mouth-puckering taste of astringent foods is mostly familiar through beverages like tea and coffee. Food sources are primarily all kinds of beans, including soybeans, along with lentils, dried peas, and other legumes. But mild astringency is present in many fruits and vegetables, including tart apples, artichokes, asparagus, bell peppers, celery, cherries, cranberries, cucumbers, figs, lemons, mushrooms, pomegranates, persimmons, potatoes, and spinach. Rye and buttermilk are notably astringent.

The sixth taste, astringent, is the least familiar to Western palates until it is pointed out as the predominant taste in tea. In Ayurveda, astringent foods extend their dry, compacting, and puckering effect to the whole body. Although medical science doesn't classify these astringent properties as an actual taste (your tongue doesn't have specific taste buds for either pungency or astringency), the natural chemicals that produce astringency are considered by Ayurveda to have health benefits: they help regulate digestion (countering diarrhea, for example) and enhance wound healing. Astringent legumes are rich in complex carbohydrates, vegetable protein, and both soluble and insoluble fiber.

Good News for Coffee Lovers

For years many people who love a strong cup of freshly brewed coffee have felt guilty about what coffee might be doing to their health. A growing body of research studies, however, now suggests that drinking up to 3 to 5 cups of coffee a day plays a potential role in preventing a range of disorders, including type 2 diabetes, Parkinson's disease, Alzheimer's disease, cancer, and cardiovascular disease.

Although researchers are still working to discover why coffee is so beneficial, they do know that it contains powerful antioxidants that help prevent free radicals from damaging bodily tissues. Coffee also contains trace minerals, including magnesium and chromium, that allow the body to make use of insulin and thus regulate blood sugar.

Choose organic coffee so you're not potentially ingesting pesticides and other toxins that may cancel out the health benefits of your morning brew. Also, steer clear of artificial sweeteners such as saccharin, aspartame, and sucralose, which contain a variety of chemicals that create toxicity in the body, according to Ayurveda.

What About Alcohol?

Although some forms of alcohol, such as red wine, have antioxidant properties, in Ayurveda any health benefits are outweighed by the negative effects of alcohol consumption. First, alcohol is high in sugar and calories, while offering relatively few nutrients (none in its pure form, as in vodka). A pint of beer or 8 ounces of wine contains about 200 calories; 1 ounce of distilled liquor has about 80 calories. The calories in alcohol can easily contribute to weight gain and obesity. When consumed in excess, alcohol also has the potential to damage every system in the body, including the central nervous system, liver, and digestive tract.

Even in moderation, alcohol interferes with the quality of sleep for some people. When you don't get enough sleep, your body decreases its production of the hormone leptin, which leads to feeling less satisfied when you eat. At the same time, a lack of sleep triggers an increase in the production of the hormone ghrelin, stimulating your appetite and making you eat more. This imbalance contributes to weight gain.

The third argument against alcohol is that it dulls awareness. This book has constantly urged you to rely on your awareness and expand it for greater joy, balance, and well-being. Alcohol runs counter to that intention because it blunts your emotions, depletes your energy, and diminishes mental clarity.

I recognize that despite these caveats, drinking is part of the everyday life of millions of people. It smooths social interactions, complements restaurant meals, and becomes the self-medication of choice at the end of a hard day. If you want to drink, the best course is to limit yourself to a glass of red wine or the equivalent—a single cocktail, a 12-ounce bottle of beer—and to have it with food. Your body will appreciate it if this consumption doesn't happen every day. Despite the traditional tolerance that doctors have shown to "having a little drink," we are just beginning to discover how to achieve optimal health and well-being. The evidence that alcohol plays a part in disease formation means that it most likely isn't part of any program for perfect health.

The Six Tastes Summarized

In order to include all six tastes in your meals, you may need to experiment with different foods and new spices. The recipes included at the end of the book offer a variety of tastes to inspire you. If you find it difficult to include all six tastes in a particular meal, at least experience each of them at some point during the day. Once you get started, you'll find it easier and easier to incorporate all six tastes.

Taste	Food Sources	Basis of Taste	Effect on Mind-Body Physiology
Sweet	*Favor:* Whole grains, fruits, starchy vegetables, and low-fat organic dairy *Reduce:* Meat (including chicken and fish), molasses, and honey *Eliminate:* Refined sugars, grains, pasta, and rice	Carbohydrates, protein, and fat	Has a soothing effect on the body. Brings about satisfaction and builds body mass.

Sour	*Favor:* Citrus fruits, berries, and tomatoes *Reduce:* Pickled and fermented foods, and alcohol	Organic acids: ascorbic acid, citric acid, acetic acid	Stimulates the appetite and aids digestion (but can be irritating to those who have heartburn).
Salty	You don't need to favor salty foods because salt is present in so many of the foods we eat. *Reduce:* Highly salted foods like potato chips, pretzels, salted meats, and processed tomato juice	Mineral salts	Enhances the appetite and makes other tastes more delicious. However, excessive salt dulls the sense of taste.
Bitter	*Favor:* All green and yellow vegetables	Alkaloids or glycosides	Detoxifying to the system. Excess intake may cause gas or indigestion.
Pungent	*Favor:* All spicy foods in small amounts, including peppers, chilies, onions, garlic, cayenne, black pepper, cloves, ginger, and mustard	Essential oils	Promotes sweating and clears the sinus passages. Stimulates metabolism.
Astringent	*Favor:* Lentils, peas, beans, green apples, berries, figs, green tea, pomegranates	Tannins	Has a drying and compacting influence on the body. Regulates digestion and helps in wound healing.

Expanded Flavors

I was born into a new era for India, immediately after the country achieved independence from the British in 1945. My parents were immensely proud to be part of this new generation, but their gaze still looked west. My father, a physician, had no patience for traditional Indian medicine. For him, Ayurveda belonged to the world of village healers and home remedies, something surpassed by advanced Western medicine.

My brother, Sanjiv, and I followed in his footsteps, both becoming Boston doctors. It took many changes, social and personal, before Ayurveda struck a chord with me. Once it did, I recognized an ancient way of living, not simply a system of medicine, and this way of living gave human beings a place in nature that was harmonious and holistic. The body wasn't a machine that you take to the doctor for repairs when a part breaks down. It was a mirror of the cosmos, its rhythms connected to the stars and the tides, its cells filled with profound intelligence, and its purpose to make daily existence joyful and productive.

Tuning in to the body isn't a casual choice in Ayurveda—it is a link to nature's deepest intelligence. As a label, "tuning in" seems too general and amorphous when it involves checking to see if anything hurts or has grown stiff. In Ayurveda, tuning in is specific. The six tastes show how precise Ayurvedic knowledge is, and they are only one frequency, so to speak, of the body's message system. Ayurveda is about the give-and-take between mind and body, preceding our modern understanding of feedback loops by many centuries. After mapping the body's messaging system in great detail, the sages of Ayurveda devised a way of life that extends everywhere. Let me show you the bigger picture of where the six tastes lead.

Flavors of Emotion

Ayurveda holds that emotions are a crucial part of the mind-body conversation. The six tastes aren't restricted to food—they are considered qualities of awareness that describe our emotions. At a deep level, we recognize this relationship because every language uses metaphors of taste to describe feelings. We are all familiar with expressions like *sweet dreams*, *salty language*, *spicy jokes*, *a bitter dispute*, and *dry wit*.

Just as it's important to include all six tastes in your meals, your brain responds to all the flavors of life, and even though bitterness and sourness aren't perceived as positive emotions, humans have evolved with a desire to experience as much of life as possible—we take the bitter with the sweet. The drama of life is played out through opposites. If someone is sweet all the time, the effect is cloying, just as eating ice cream all day would be. A touch of sourness adds depth, but too much makes us grimace. Don't overemphasize any emotional flavor, but by the same token don't completely neglect any either. Every flavor has its place in the metabolizing of experience, and cultivating a balance of all the flavors adds richness to your experience.

Emotions: The Flavors of Life

Taste	Balanced	Out of Balance
Sweet	Nurturing	Cloying
Sour	Stimulating	Caustic
Salty	Hearty	Aggravated
Bitter	Energized	Resentful
Pungent	Passionate	Hostile
Astringent	Witty	Cynical

Food and the Rainbow of Colors

Along with including the six tastes in every meal, filling your plate with the colors of the rainbow provides visual appeal. What pleases the eye pleases the body as a whole. Close your eyes and imagine that you are on a sunny Caribbean beach. Beside the sparkling blue water a picnic has been laid out, an exotic one. Instead of china you are eating off banana leaves. The meal is a visual feast: grilled fish topped with bright orange mangos, fragrant white rice with shaved coconut, and vivid pink watermelon with lime wedges. As you visualize this meal, you are likely to find that your appetite is stimulated by the images and that your expectation is of a happy experience. These messages are coursing throughout your body.

You can create the same messages in real time with actual food. It takes only a few minutes to add vibrant color to a meal with parsley, mint, and other herbs, a wedge of lemon or lime, and/or a dab of bottled chutney—restaurants devote considerable ingenuity to making their presentations sell the food as much as its flavors. Ayurveda looks upon color as a kind of flavor on its own. In your mind's eye, see a white china plate filled with steamed fish, cauliflower, and rice. The fact that everything is white all but screams blandness, even though the tastes on the tongue are varied. On its own, however, white is the color of purity; the key is to offer it in combination with other colors.

Here are a few suggestions for adding vibrancy to the color palette of your meals. In Ayurveda, an ideal spectrum would include every color.

Red	Raspberries, apples, cherries, strawberries, pomegranates, tomatoes, watermelon, pink grapefruit, papayas, red bell peppers, chili peppers
Orange	Oranges, melons, mangos, apricots, sweet potatoes, carrots
Yellow	Lemons, bananas, pineapple, peaches, yellow squash, corn, yellow bell peppers
Green	Kiwi, apples, limes, green grapes, spinach, lettuce, Swiss chard, arugula, kale, collard greens, broccoli, artichokes, asparagus, celery, avocados, zucchini, Brussels sprouts, green peas

Blue and Purple	Blueberries, purple grapes, "red" cabbage, beets, eggplant, plums
White	Pears, coconuts, onions, garlic, cauliflower, parsnips, rutabagas

Ayurveda also sees a nutritional connection here. Foods with deep, rich colors are leaders in antioxidants and contain many phytonutrients, those derived from plants, that boost immunity and enhance health. The best recent research suggests that the most healing foods are those containing potent concentrations of the plant-based compounds that are responsible for flavor and color. The six tastes are well coordinated with these compounds.

A drawback of breaking nutrition down into its chemical components is that we don't actually experience phytonutrients. It's unlikely that you will say to a friend, "I just had the most delicious lycopenes for lunch," or "That was the best flavonoid I ever tasted!" I'm including this information on phytonutrients because knowledge is power, but I encourage you to focus on making your meals a rich experience. By enjoying the sensory pleasures of eating with awareness, you will nourish yourself more completely than any nutritional chart could ever achieve.

Here are a few of the health-enhancing phytonutrients contained in fresh fruits, vegetables, spices, and herbs.

Phytochemical	Actions	Sources	Tastes
Flavonoids	Antioxidant, anticarcinogenic, protect against heart disease	Onions, broccoli, red grapes, apples, cherries, citrus fruits, berries, tomatoes	Sour, pungent, sweet
Phenolic compounds	Antioxidant, inhibit cancerous changes	Nuts, berries, green tea	Astringent, sour, sweet

Phytochemical	Actions	Sources	Tastes
Sulfides	Antioxidant, anticarcinogenic, inhibit blood clotting	Garlic, onions, chives	Pungent
Lycopenes	Antioxidant, anticarcinogenic	Tomatoes, red grapefruit	Sour
Isothiocyanates	Inhibit cancer growth	Broccoli, cabbage, cauliflower	Astringent
Isoflavones	Block hormonally stimulated cancers, lower cholesterol levels	Soybeans, soy-derived foods, garbanzo beans, pinto beans, navy beans	Sweet, astringent
Anthocyanins	Antioxidant, lower cholesterol, stimulate immunity	Berries, cherries, grapes, currants	Sweet, sour
Terpenoids	Antioxidant, antibacterial, prevent stomach ulcers	Peppers, cinnamon, horseradish, rosemary, thyme, turmeric	Pungent, bitter
Lignans	Anticarcinogenic, lower cholesterol and blood pressure	Flaxseed, sesame seed, wheat bran, olives	Astringent, sweet
Coumestans	Anticarcinogenic	Clover, alfalfa, and soybean sprouts; split peas, pinto beans, lima beans	Bitter, astringent
Phthalides	Lower blood pressure and cholesterol, anticarcinogenic	Celery, carrots, parsley, parsnips, fennel	Astringent, bitter, sweet

Spices for Wellness

Before pharmaceuticals arrived on the scene, traditional medicine relied on herbs, spices, and other natural products for their healing properties. Ayurveda is no exception, and research studies, primarily from India, continue to explore these remedies. The medicinal properties of most drugs cannot be identified in advance with rough chemical analysis, so drug companies still comb the medicine chest of natural remedies to find new cures.

This book isn't concerned with remedies, but since Ayurveda is holistic, many foods are recommended that have healing properties. What follows are a few spices and other strong flavorings with notes about their potential benefits in keeping you well. Spices are intensely flavorful, and therefore they send strong messages to your body (without adding calories). Although researchers have isolated the active ingredients in some herbs and spices and made them available in pill form, they have been stripped from their natural setting and are definitely less enjoyable than savoring whole foods prepared with fresh spices and herbs.

Note: The benefits mentioned under each spice come from the Ayurvedic tradition; no medical claims are being made. At the Chopra Center our emphasis is on creating wellness. In the presence of disease symptoms, which Ayurveda considers an advanced stage of imbalance, Western medicine is often the most effective approach since it specializes in the outbreak of disease. Ayurveda specializes in maintaining long-term balance and wellness, a different approach.

Ginger

Ginger is a pungent, aromatic spice that has long been used in traditional healing systems to improve digestion and alleviate nausea, intestinal gas, and menstrual cramps. Ayurveda recommends using the fresh root over dried powdered ginger. Researchers have found that ginger contains anti-inflammatory phytonutrients known as *gingerols*, as well as strong antioxidant and antibacterial properties. Here are a few of the recent findings about ginger's potential benefits:

- Consuming ginger on a regular basis can help reduce pain levels and swelling in people with osteoarthritis or rheumatoid arthritis.
- Researchers have found that ginger contains specific compounds that may bind to serotonin receptors in the brain, which could help alleviate anxiety.
- Ginger is effective in preventing the symptoms of motion sickness, including nausea, dizziness, and vomiting.
- Small doses of ginger can also help relieve nausea and vomiting related to pregnancy, without the adverse side effects associated with antinausea drugs.
- Studies suggest that ginger may also be helpful in stabilizing metabolism, including reducing the risk of diabetes.
- Ginger may inhibit the growth of some kinds of human cancer cells, including colorectal cancer cells.

There are many ways to enjoy ginger, and I've included recipes for ginger tea and other dishes. It's better to use fresh ginger rather than the dried powdered form of the spice—it will have superior flavor and greater levels of gingerol and other anti-inflammatory compounds. If you use dried ginger, try to find an organically grown product that has not been irradiated.

Another Ayurvedic tip: Drink ginger tea or warm water before each meal. This will improve your digestion and decrease the tendency to overeat.

Turmeric

In Ayurveda this beautiful yellow spice is a pharmacy unto itself. To begin with, research has found that turmeric contains potent anti-inflammatory and antioxidant properties—these are valuable given the suspicious connection between low-level chronic inflammation and many lifestyle disorders. Here are a few other possible uses:

- Turmeric has a protective effect on the liver and can help reduce elevated blood cholesterol levels.
- In the treatment of arthritis, turmeric, when used alone or in combination with other compounds, can reduce pain and stiffness.
- Several studies in animals have demonstrated that turmeric can prevent or inhibit the development of certain cancer cells.
- Turmeric has a soothing effect on digestion and can help reduce the risk of ulcers and upset stomach.
- As a natural antibiotic agent, turmeric can inhibit the growth of bacteria, yeast, and viruses under laboratory conditions.

One of the primary active ingredients in turmeric is known as curcumin, which is not easily absorbed by the body, but another chemical, the piperine in black pepper, can increase the absorption of curcumin. Turmeric and pepper are components of most curry powder blends. Studies by epidemiologists indicate that in India, where curry is the mainstay of everyday diets, the rates of Alzheimer's disease are among the lowest in the world. In the population of 70- to 79-year-olds, the rate is less than 25 percent of that in the United States. Although a lower life expectancy and death from other causes play important parts, some researchers hypothesize that the anti-inflammatory and antioxidant properties of a compound like curcumin may be a major factor in preventing Alzheimer's. You can enjoy turmeric in soups, sautéed vegetables, and other dishes where brilliant color and mild spiciness add a new dimension.

Cinnamon

Cinnamon is a sweet, warming, pungent spice derived from the inner bark of the cinnamon tree. Since ancient times cinnamon has been used to increase energy and treat colds, indigestion, and cramps. While there are approximately one hundred varieties of *cinnamonum verum* trees, the most common variety in the United States is commonly referred to as cassia. Cinnamon is a powerful antioxidant and contains compounds that decrease inflammation and fight against bacteria, viruses, and fungi. Cinnamon may help reduce chronic inflammation, which is linked with neurological disorders such as Alzheimer's disease, Parkinson's disease, multiple sclerosis, and meningitis. Researchers continue to add to a growing body of findings. Here are some of the most recent discoveries:

- A number of studies indicate that cassia cinnamon may be helpful in treating type 2 diabetes because it lowers blood sugar levels and increases insulin production.
- Cinnamon contains an anti-inflammatory compound known as *cinnamaldehyde*, which helps prevent unhealthy clumping of blood platelets.
- Studies have found that cinnamon can help reduce the LDL cholesterol level and decrease the risk of heart disease.
- Cinnamon decreases the proliferation of leukemia and lymphoma cancer cells under laboratory conditions.
- When combined with honey, cinnamon can reduce arthritic pain.
- The fragrance of cinnamon can help improve cognitive function, including focus, memory, and visual-motor speed.

When you buy cinnamon, whether in stick or powder form, smell it to make sure that it has a strong, sweet fragrance.

Peppers

Used in many of the world's cuisines, both spicy and sweet peppers contain many phytochemicals with antioxidant properties. (Although they share the same name, black peppercorns aren't from the same family as chilies, bell peppers, and related fruits.) Fresh peppers come in a variety of colors, including red, yellow, green, and purple. Each color is associated with a different family of phytochemicals and other nutrients. Red peppers, for example, are a rich source of lycopenes, lutein (which is beneficial for eye health), beta-carotene, and vitamins B_6, C, and A.

Spicy peppers such as jalapeños and habaneros contain high levels of an enzyme called capsaicin, a natural antioxidant that makes you break into a sweat and tear up when you take a bite. Researchers have found that spicy peppers may increase metabolism and curb the appetite, benefits that can help with weight loss. Here are some of the recent findings about capsaicin (which is found only in tiny quantities in bell peppers and other sweet kinds):

- Capsaicin helps reduce pain by depleting a chemical called substance P, which transmits pain signals to the brain. Studies have found that capsaicin provides pain relief from migraine and sinus headaches.
- Studies in animals have found that capsaicin can be effective in killing cancer cells in the pancreas, prostate, and lungs.
- Capsaicin may help prevent cardiovascular disease by reducing cholesterol and triglycerides and preventing unhealthy blood clotting.
- Peppers contain antibacterial properties that help fight chronic sinus infections.

As the American diet becomes more diverse, including dishes from all over the world, cooks are using peppers in salads, salsa, guacamole, and curries. Try to eat a variety of peppers so that you get a wide range of the phytonutrients they offer.

Garlic

Garlic is native to central Asia but was also well known in ancient China, Greece, and Egypt. For many centuries this pungent herb has been a staple in the Mediterranean region, valued for both medicinal and culinary purposes. It has a long-standing reputation as an effective treatment for relieving lung congestion and arthritic stiffness and pain. In traditional healing garlic has also been used to calm anxiety, promote regular menstruation in women, and improve libido in men. Garlic oil is applied topically to soothe sore muscles and accelerate the healing of wounds.

Thousands of scientific studies have been published on this complex botanical ally, which contains almost two hundred different chemical components. Most of them haven't been carefully researched yet. Most research to date has focused on allicin, a phytochemical in garlic that has various healing properties. Here is what the most recent scientific understanding of garlic reveals:

- Raw garlic has potent antibacterial, antifungal, and antiviral properties. It can help strengthen the immune system, prevent the common cold, and treat fungal and yeast infections.
- Garlic may reduce the risk of some cancers, including breast, prostate, stomach, and colon cancer. Researchers found that people who eat more than six garlic cloves a week had a 30 percent lower rate of colorectal cancer and a 50 percent lower rate of stomach cancer than non–garlic eaters.
- Garlic helps relieve sinus congestion.
- Some studies indicate that garlic can help reduce blood cholesterol levels, though further research is needed to confirm these findings and determine which forms of garlic are most beneficial.

- Studies have found that that regular consumption of garlic helps prevent atherosclerosis and heart disease by decreasing plaque and calcium deposits in coronary arteries, reducing unhealthy blood clotting, and improving blood circulation.

Keep in mind that when garlic is cooked or dried, it loses most of its medicinal benefits. For this reason, garlic pills don't offer the same health value as eating fresh, raw garlic. If you love garlicky food but don't like the effect it has on your breath, one possible remedy is parsley, chewed after the meal or taken in pill form, easily found in health food stores.

The Earliest Prevention

By breaking each disease down into its components, scientific medicine has achieved an astonishing sophistication. Within days after a new strain of flu breaks out, the virus that causes it can be analyzed. Cancers are being tracked down to the molecular level and typed according to the patient's genome.

But Ayurveda holds that advanced diagnosis—which is the great strength of scientific medicine—comes into play at the end of a long string of events. Before any symptoms appear, the stage where drugs and surgery are forced to step in, the body's own healing system has reached a critical stage of breakdown. Breakdown is the result of feedback loops that are overloaded through some kind of drastic imbalance. Imbalance begins at a subtle level that makes itself known through signals of comfort and discomfort. So the long chain of events that culminates with illness actually begins with everyday choices that either help your body remain in balance or throw it out of balance.

This simple logic isn't denied by modern medicine. But physicians are trained as interventionists who spring into action after the damage is too advanced for the body to take care of itself. There is no training in the predisease state, although in the past two decades the overwhelming role that prevention can play has begun to make an impression on the mainstream medical community.

Ayurveda keeps its sights fixed on how to create the good life, following practices that merge mind and body. On a daily basis you should choose the most nourishing input, whether your choice is based on Ayurveda or on principles couched in the language of feedback loops. A balanced, harmonious lifestyle represents the earliest prevention program. Here's a quick summary of the lifestyle I've recommended in this book.

Long Before Illness Appears, Your Best Choices:

Eat natural, whole foods.
Follow your body's signals of hunger and satiation.
Tune in to sensations of discomfort and heed them.
Pay attention to daily biorhythms, particularly sleep.
Remain in a state of restful alertness.
Promote energy and lightness in your diet and also in your choice of exercise.
Consciously deal with stress levels.
Have a vision of well-being and follow it.

The best way to prevent illness is to live so harmoniously that the subtle precursors of disease (i.e., early imbalances) don't gain a toehold in the mind-body system. That's the assumption followed by Ayurveda, and even though its principles were laid down more than two thousand years before the rise of science, with no technical understanding of homeostasis or feedback loops in the brain, today's best knowledge about wellness and illness comes remarkably close to the major themes of Ayurveda.

The first signs of imbalance aren't mysterious; we're all well acquainted with them, with a host of low-grade symptoms such as fatigue, lack of energy, insomnia, susceptibility to colds and flu, heartburn, headaches, digestive problems, ill-defined aches and pains, depression, and anxiety. Being low-grade, not yet rising to the level of serious symptoms (most of the time), these peripheral signals don't mean much in Western medicine unless they persist. Even then, it's assumed that peripheral discomforts aren't as serious as full-blown diseases.

Ayurveda takes the opposite view, seeing early imbalance as the first link in the chain of events that will lead eventually to a full-blown disease. This perspective has been rapidly gaining ground in scientific medicine, however, once researchers realized that genetic changes linked to diabetes, autism, depression, schizophrenia, and Alzheimer's disease—just to mention a few prominent disorders—crop up years and sometimes decades before symptoms appear. We also realize that lifestyle choices have long-term consequences in changing genetic output. Genes don't simply turn on or off like a light switch but work on a sliding scale like a dimmer switch or rheostat.

That's why the daily input entering the mind-body system is so important. The body is built like a sand dune, one grain at a time, not like a wall, one brick at a time. So each day is a microcosm of your whole life—what you eat, think, feel, and do is foretelling your future. The experience of harmonious living today foretells a harmonious future, which is different from living any way you want to until the day when bad things start to happen, at which point you must scurry to make up for your past. Sometimes that isn't possible.

Can Ayurveda solve the problem of noncompliance? I think so. After decades of public health campaigns, Americans continue to be sedentary and to eat the wrong diet. One of the main reasons is the climate of fear surrounding cancer, heart disease, stroke, Alzheimer's disease, and other major diseases. These are largely disorders of middle to old age, and people fear them so much because they belong to a frightening image of overall decline. Fear-based motivation rarely works over the long haul. On a day-to-day basis, people won't comply out of anxiety.

Ayurveda turns the situation around with its focus on early imbalances. These are not frightening. Quite the opposite. Living a harmonious, balanced life adds to your happiness and staves off the specter of what might befall you in your declining years. By being in balance, you don't have to decline. The "new old age" has already replaced the worst assumptions about old people sitting uselessly in rocking chairs, lonely and unnoticed. The baby boom generation sees seventy as late middle age, and one survey that asked when old age begins found that the average answer was eighty-five. The best way to live a long, active life is to have that expectation in mind.

The key is to find a lifestyle that makes you happy at twenty, thirty, fifty, and eighty. I believe that Ayurveda lays a good basis for such a lifestyle. If you add another element, you can make your entire life span a rising arc, with no fear of decline. That added element is higher consciousness, which we are ready to explore to the fullest. Awareness eating is just one application of awareness—a wider horizon opens when you discover that awareness holds the key to the higher states of mental and spiritual fulfillment.

PART TWO

RAISING YOUR CONSCIOUSNESS

The Joy of Awareness

Power Points

- When you eat, either you are aware of what you are doing or you have blanked out, unconsciously taking in your food.
- Many people eat unconsciously, which is why their eating is out of control. You can only control what you're aware of. When you eat unconsciously, you go blank and don't realize what you're doing. Going blank is a choice—you don't have to do it.
- Mindfulness provides a simple way to tune in to your brain, which is sending you four kinds of messages: sensations, images, feelings, and thoughts (SIFT).
- The joy of awareness dawns when you can escape the prison of conditioning. Awareness is all about restoring your freedom to choose what you want instead of what your past imposes on you.

Several times I've underlined the point that you can't control what you're not aware of. For me this was a surprising lesson at first, because I overestimated my own awareness, not in all areas but in several. One was my medical career. For years I strove for success through self-discipline, the kind that got me up at five in the morning so that I could make the rounds at two local hospitals before driving to my private practice, where my patient roster ran into the thousands. Success came, but not the feeling of satisfaction that is supposed to be one of the great rewards of success.

Then one day a wise friend said, "You know, I think you've got willpower down. Have you considered acceptance? You don't have to keep running all the time." He might have added a few more things that are crucial to finding satisfaction, such as showing gratitude and learning to live in the present.

I had a lot to learn about the art of living. It came to me in the end—or so I hope—and I'd like to spend the rest of this book showing you what that means. I'm disturbed and also moved by the fact that millions of people have become unconscious of what they're doing with their lives. Happiness isn't meant to be so elusive. It's the natural by-product of waking up to who you are and why you are here. You can find out those things only through expanded awareness, but expanded awareness depends on something that comes first: the courage to see your situation without denial or giving in to the temptation to be unconscious.

Let's start with the way that unconscious behavior applies to overweight, because that's the situation in which readers of this book find themselves. Hopefully you've already begun to change, applying the action steps of awareness eating. But awareness can take you much further, as we'll see.

The Missing Element

Alison is in her early thirties and came for a consultation because she was gaining weight but had no idea why. In her own mind, she was doing everything right.

"I was brought up to eat healthily, and I still do," she said. "When my daughter came along—she's four now—I became extra careful during my pregnancy, cutting out alcohol and junk food entirely. I kept that up after she was born, but my hormones must have changed, because I'm twenty-five pounds heavier than I've ever been."

I asked her if the weight gain started soon after her baby was born. Alison thought for a moment but wasn't sure.

"It was like two years went by, and suddenly none of my clothes fit anymore," she said.

We talked about the changes that happened in her life after becoming a new mother. She couldn't afford to stay home with her child, and going back to work so soon after giving birth put new pressures on Alison that she hadn't experienced before. There was some strain in her marriage, too, since her husband felt that Alison was putting all her attention on the baby and had less interest in him, particularly when it came to the bedroom. Exhaustion was her main defense, but the strain was still present four years later. She had a lot to face, and often that's a motivation to bury some things, for fear of being overwhelmed.

I suggested that we postpone any medical tests for the moment (which were likely to be inconclusive, since hormonal imbalance, if we found any, could be the result of gaining weight, not the cause). Instead, I asked Alison to go home and keep a daily record of everything she ate. For each item she was to write down what she ate and how much.

When we met again a week later, she looked chagrined. It turned out that she was eating more than she had imagined—although not that much.

I told Alison that studies where overweight people carefully count calories reveal that they are consuming more than they thought, while at the same time they overestimate how much physical activity they are getting. "When you eat more than you think and are active less than you think, you're going to gain weight," I said.

"You could keep a diary of your daily food intake," I said, "but most people give up after a while. It's a tedious task, and they lose motivation. I think your whole problem can be solved by being aware of your eating."

Alison was surprised and intrigued. Most overeaters are eating in a state of unawareness. They go blank, and it doesn't take more than a few times before those blank spots add up to excess weight. Instead of being vigilant about how much food one eats (no one can keep track if they've gone blank to begin with), you can use the mind-body connection and stay conscious while you eat. Here are the most likely suspects when you investigate those moments of going blank.

Your Most Likely Blank Spots

Racing through a meal; not really tasting what you're eating
Snacking while watching TV
Taking second helpings even after you're full
Automatically finishing your entire plate of food
Eating when you're tired
Eating when you're stressed

I told Alison that because she considered herself a healthy eater, just being aware of these vulnerable spots would probably be all that she needed. So far, it's worked out that way. Alison recognized one major blank spot, which was tension at the dinner table between her and her husband. Both had retreated emotionally, which never solves underlying tensions. Unable to enjoy her meal in a relaxed, apprecia-tive way, Alison still wanted to feel some kind of satisfaction, which came from eating more.

Many people will find it threatening to look at their eating habits only to discover that there's a lot more to examine. They'd prefer to keep eating in a separate compartment away from emotional or re-lationship issues. But if you feel this kind of uneasiness, I'd urge you to change your perspective. Denial and avoidance are ways of being unconscious. What you are unconscious of can't be changed; in fact, with time the only thing that happens is that buried issues get worse. As one therapist remarked to me, "What you resist persists."

Alison was fortunate, because she was basically asking for permission to wake up. She didn't want to be unconscious. Having seen how uncomfortable she felt at the dinner table, she took heart and began to face the issue, which began by admitting her discomfort to her husband. No surprise, he felt much the same way on his side of the dinner table. Both of them wanted to discuss the problems in their marriage, and the good news is that once their feelings were out in the open, they felt better. Anxiety and resentment began to lessen— with the help of a marriage counselor at the beginning—and Alison had less and less reason to overeat. Her life was coming back under control, and almost as a side effect she began to lose weight.

Family Dynamics

Alison's story is a reminder that few of us eat alone, and we certainly didn't learn how to eat by ourselves. Every child develops eating habits as part of a family. One of the main reasons for continuing your bad eating habits today is also family. Stop for a moment and consider a typical scene at your dinner table. What's the mood? How much are the family members interacting? Whatever your answer is, there's a lot going on at the table besides passing the salt and putting food in your stomach.

Studies have shown that behavior is contagious; it spreads from person to person like an invisible virus. If you have someone in your family who likes to exercise, or even a friend, it's much more likely that you will exercise, too. On the other hand, if you have family and friends who are obese, your risk of obesity goes up, even though you may not consciously realize what's happening. As it relates to eating, the viral spread of behavior works either positively or negatively.

Quiz:
Your Family at the Table

Listed here are two categories of "infectious" behavior. The first category contains positive influences regarding eating; the second contains negative influences. Check each item that typically applies to you and your family when you eat together. Use the past *two weeks* as your time frame.

Positive Influences

___ We enjoy being together and create a happy mood.

___ The atmosphere is relaxed.

___ The pace of eating is relaxed.

___ No one is in a rush to leave. We often linger at the table after we've finished eating.

___ Appreciation is expressed to the cook.

___ We say a blessing over the food.

___ We eat with relish. No one balks at certain foods or complains about what they're eating.

___ We realize as a family that healthy eating is enjoyable.

___ We don't snack before or after meals.

___ Portions are moderate. No one sticks out by eating too much or too little.

___ We are open about our eating habits. If someone is habitually overeating, it can be brought to their attention without hurting their feelings.

___ We pay full attention to the meal. The TV isn't on in the background.

Score: _____

Negative Influences

___ When we eat together, we tend to take each other for granted.

There's not much talk. One or two family members barely participate.

___ The atmosphere is neutral or tense. Personal remarks are made.

___ The pace of eating is fast so that everyone can go back to what they want to do.

___ As soon as the food is finished, everyone leaves the table. There's no lingering.

___ Quite often the cook isn't praised, or somebody mutters a few perfunctory words.

___ We don't say a blessing or give thanks over the food.

___ Someone complains about what's on their plate or says that the cooking isn't good.

___ There's no discussion about healthy eating.

___ At least one or two of us snack before or after meals.

___ Portions are big. Even so, somebody usually wants second helpings.

___ We don't talk about our eating habits. If someone is habitually overeating, they don't welcome it if anyone else notices. How each person eats is their own business.

___ We don't really pay that much attention to what we're eating. The TV is sometimes on in the background.

Score: _____

Rating Yourself

If you checked *8 to 12 positive items*, your family dynamic is healthy. Eating dinner together is a complete and satisfying experience. Because you bond so well, you are "infecting" each other with positive behavior, and your efforts to make everyone's eating even healthier will be welcomed—congratulations.

If you checked *3 to 7 positive items*, you are having a good experience at the dinner table. Your family is likely to be supportive if you change your eating habits to lose weight or simply to eat more healthily. (Fewer than 3 positive items means that you likely fall into the negative group of influences.)

If you checked *8 to 12 negative items*, your family dynamic isn't good around the table. It is unlikely that you can smoothly change your eating habits, either to lose weight or to eat more healthily. You need to stop the "infection" of bad habits by working on yourself. Start following the principles of awareness eating and gradually move your family in the right direction as far as introducing a healthy diet. The best way to induce change is away from the table—there will be too much resistance if you spring any changes without notice. Sit down and talk about ways to eat better that everyone can agree on, even if the changes are small. Meanwhile, gain the benefits of working on yourself. The family setting may not be ideal, but that shouldn't stop you.

If you checked *3 to 7 negative items*, your family dynamic is stuck in bad habits and unconscious behaviors. The situation probably doesn't feel that serious to you, but even neutral eating can't be called satisfying. The dinner table at your house is likely to be a place where a truce has been drawn. One or more family members aren't happy being there, or a general air of indifference may prevail. The good news is that you have a good chance of coaxing everyone else to join you either to lose weight or to eat more healthily. Your meals need to be more satisfying, and there's lots of room for that. Consult the Ayurvedic advice about making meals tastier and more vibrant.

If you have stubborn eaters who are completely resistant to change, be strategic. Invite them to join you in your new regimen. Give them a week or two to see how much you like your new way of eating. If you still meet with strong resistance, tell anyone in the family who is sixteen or older that they must take some responsibility for what they eat. This could involve several choices:

- Give them some printed information about healthy eating (e.g., a book or Internet article), making it clear that you want to sit down and discuss the long-term risks of an unhealthy diet.

- Negotiate terms. Sit down and set some limits on the intake of fats, sugar, salt, and overall calories. For everything that gets reduced, promise that their food will continue to taste good, and if it doesn't, you will be willing to offer a more pleasing substitute.

- If you hit a wall discussing a better way to eat, tell the person that they will be cooking for themselves, without extra money to spend on junk food and meals at chains like McDonald's and Wendy's. They are expected to keep eating with the rest of the family.

- It may not seem feasible to reach the stage where all twelve positive items are part of your family's experience, but they are achievable. The first step is to make yourself aware of what is going on around the dinner table and then diplomatically help others become as aware as you are, without judgment, blame, or complaint.

You Have a Right to Be Aware

As much as you will benefit from being more aware, others don't see it that way. Their agenda is to keep you unaware. The food industry is often blamed—and rightfully so—for stuffing excess sugar, salt, and fat into its processed products. But what is more pernicious is its attack on awareness. Foods are deliberately manufactured to encourage robotic eating, such as "munching rhythm," where the teasing taunt made famous by Lay's potato chips comes true: "Bet you can't eat just one." The snack industry and fast-food chains want you to obey the automatic hunger response created by too much salt and fat, which are appetite stimulants. In addition, they pour on the same three tastes—salty, sweet, and sour—that trigger salivation. You'll recall that Ayurveda considers these tastes the ones most likely to lead to imbalances.

Eating snacks and fast food depends on the public obeying unconscious cues, and not just in the area of tastes. Becoming fixated on these foods happens when you aren't even aware. To prove this to yourself, try a simple mind-body experiment. Close your eyes and see a lemon in your mind's eye. Now mentally take a knife and cut the lemon in half. See a drop of lemon juice coming out. As you do, what happens? Almost everyone starts to salivate. Just the sight of a lemon is enough to bypass your higher brain. Junk food becomes addictive because you have memories of all the salty, sweet, and sour food that stimulated you in the past. The food industry counts on those memories to be triggered when you look at tempting pictures of juicy burgers, hear the crunch of potato chips in a TV commercial, or watch the expression of semiorgasmic delight when a model bites into a chocolate bar.

You must reclaim your right to be aware. If you don't, an avalanche of suggestive selling will keep coaxing you to go blank. It doesn't take many blank moments to lead to extra pounds. A child who has been goaded by Saturday morning TV to demand a meal at McDonald's would consume 1,842 calories in a large combo meal. A Big Mac alone is 700 calories, more than half of what a small child needs per day. An unconscious craving for sweet, salty, fatty food is being reinforced, while at the same time the amount of calories in the combo meal is enough for a 175-pound adult male who ate nothing else that day. (In an eye-opening 2004 documentary, *Super Size Me*, filmmaker Morgan Spurlock gained nearly 25 pounds by existing entirely on McDonald's meals for a month. As he put on the pounds, Spurlock found his health deteriorating as his cholesterol and blood pressure skyrocketed, while at the same time his libido crashed. Although a stunt, *Super Size Me* struck close to home for many, since it was a fast-motion version of what millions of Americans are doing to their bodies.)

The policy shift to serve McDonald's in schools as a cost-cutting measure is shameful, even more so when the same unhealthy stuff is sold in hospitals. The right to be aware is yours to take back. The solution is to eat mindfully. *Mindfulness* originated as a Buddhist term and now has become popular in the West. It means that you notice what you are doing, thinking, and feeling. I've found it useful to adapt the acronym SIFT, proposed by the innovative psychiatrist and writer Dr. Daniel Siegel. It covers the four things that the mind is aware of at any given moment:

S = Sensations

I = Images

F = Feelings

T = Thoughts

Right now, your awareness is focused on one of these mental events. A bodily sensation is present, carrying messages of comfort or discomfort. Or a picture in your mind is showing you an image, which will be pleasant or unpleasant. You could also be experiencing a feeling (mood, emotion), which will be positive or negative. Finally, your mind may be occupied by thinking, and like the preceding events, thoughts can be pleasant or unpleasant.

I'm emphasizing the pleasant/unpleasant duality, because when you blank out while eating, you are avoiding the unpleasant side of SIFT and trying to numb yourself instead. Going unconscious for a moment is the same as tuning out, and we've all learned to tune out things we don't want to see, hear, feel, or think about.

When you decide to stop tuning out, you can be mindful instead. The enemies of mindfulness are well known:

Denial: You refuse to look at the problem.
Distraction: You find a diversion to take your mind off the problem.
Forgetfulness: You don't remember that the problem exists.
Numbness: You can't feel anything, so there must not be a problem.

One or more of these mechanisms takes over during unconscious eating. The inability to know when your stomach is full—one of the most common situations with overweight people—is a form of numbness. Going numb is never a solution, and even when someone acts oblivious to being obese, for example, there is another layer of the mind crying out for help and an even deeper layer where the solution exists. These deeper layers come to light simply by being mindful, because, rest assured, they want to be heard.

The things you tune out are still there. What you've deprived yourself of is the opportunity to make them better as connected to eating. Being mindful is effective in keeping the mind-body connection intact. The most basic kind of mindfulness is easy to attain and can be done at any time during your day.

Exercise:
How to Be Mindful

Find a room where you can be quiet and alone. Sit with your back straight and your feet planted apart on the floor. Put your hands on your knees and close your eyes. When you feel relaxed and ready, easily tune in to what is happening inside you. Let your awareness travel to each of the following areas.

Sensations: Notice how your body feels.

Images: Notice the fleeting images in your mind's eye.

Feelings: Notice any emotions that come up. Sense your overall mood.

Thoughts: Watch the thoughts that come and go.

Take a minute for each area before you open your eyes. Don't react to what you become aware of. Simply observe, without judgment and without trying to change anything. Being an observer is the same as getting out of the way, and when you get out of the way, you give the mind-body connection space to rest and readjust.

This exercise is an adaptation of the techniques that Dr. Siegel has employed with impressive effectiveness. His therapeutic mode is also mind-body relevant, specifically targeting each area of the brain by connecting it with discomfort, tightness, or numbness in the body. By being mindful of these symptoms, he can lead the patient to reactivate the specific area of the brain that has become underused or deficient. Attention is powerful in every way when you are aware of what you should focus on, and your body will tell you where to go. The exercise I've just recommended is quiet but not passive. You are waking up to reality "in here."

I realize that people will get anxious about tuning in to painful memories, feelings, and sensations. When you're overweight, just the thought of paying more attention to your body doesn't sound appealing. But mindfulness isn't about getting down on yourself, facing unpleasant truths, or entering into the blame game. It's about the joy of being aware. So many of the best things in life slip by when you aren't aware, and when you wake up, your whole experience of life is heightened. You find yourself accessing inner powers that were hidden from view. Creativity requires awareness. So does finding the solution to any problem.

Relating to how you eat, there are many steps in awareness that don't involve any kind of painful adjustment, as follows:

Action Step:
12 Ways to Eat Mindfully

Any action that brings your attention to the act of eating helps break the spell of going blank. This applies to what you're putting into your mouth as well as behavioral habits like how quickly you eat. Look over the following list and begin to adopt each tip. Take them one at a time, beginning with the changes that would most benefit your eating habits. (Note: Several items are summarized from previous topics—they reappear in the light of being mindful.)

1. Eat only when you feel hungry. Notice and feel your hunger. This is the basis of conscious eating.

2. To encourage your full attention, always sit down when eating your meal in settled surroundings without distractions.

3. Start with a moderate portion of food, such as half a plate. When that's finished, sit for a moment to see how hungry you may still feel. Drink a little water before taking more food.

4. Appreciate the taste of each bite by lingering over it, putting your attention on the flavor, and chewing a little more than you usually do. In other words, make taste an experience all its own.

5. Be aware that appetite is stoked by fatty, salty, and sweet tastes. Appetite is suppressed with bitter foods. Try sipping some club soda with a dash of Angostura bitters before you eat (bottled tonic water is bitter but contains too much sugar).

6. Remove the skin from chicken and the fat from all meat before you sit down to eat. In a restaurant, set these unwanted things aside on your bread plate or ask the waiter to remove them.

7. Eat at the slowest pace that feels comfortable. A moderate pace will promote optimal digestion. Don't fill your fork or spoon until you've swallowed the bite you're eating.

8. If you're a fast eater, especially if you bolt your food while talk-

ing, take small portions before you sit down. (You're going so quickly that you will hardly notice how much is on the plate.)

9. If you know you are prone to impulsive eating that gets worse as the meal continues, tell the others at the table how much you intend to eat, then keep your word. (But don't ask to be reminded. The point is to monitor your own eating, not to have others do it for you.)

10. In a restaurant, have your server immediately box the food you aren't going to eat. Don't leave it on the plate to be pecked at until it's all gone.

11. If ordering dessert, ask for half of it to be put immediately into a take-home box. Give the box as a gift to someone else at the table.

12. Fill your stomach only two-thirds of the way to feeling full (the best gauge is to eat two-thirds of your normal filling portion). Send your plate away or get up from the table at that point. Notice that you can feel comfortable in leaving a small empty space in your stomach.

The Prison of Conditioning

When you stop blanking out, you can bring more awareness to how you eat. At the same time you are beginning to break free of your old conditioning. Nothing is more crucial. Finding more freedom opens up the real joy of awareness. Without knowing it, you have been living inside a prison that has no visible walls—the confines of your cell derive entirely from the habits and conditioning of your mind. You aren't to blame for living within unnecessary limitations. But at the same time, only you hold the key to freedom. It, too, is invisible. The key is to shift from being unconscious to being aware.

I've been guiding you through that shift by showing you how to change your story. Here I'd like to outline the rewards of breaking out of your hidden limitations. Conditioning is different from going blank—it's how you've trained yourself to be. As an illustration, I can think of two patients who approached their weight problem differently. Cheryl has been carrying extra weight for as long as she can remember. When I asked her about her childhood, she didn't open up about being teased or lectures from her mother or her deep disappointment that boys didn't pay attention to her.

Even though she is 80 pounds overweight at age forty, and feeling miserable about it, Cheryl has put up lots of barriers. She never uses the word *fat*, but instead refers to herself as "a big woman." If it is pointed out that she might be eating too much (which seems obvious), she instantly becomes defensive. She is a bundle of conditioned responses; there are thick walls around her that she can't see. Even though she thinks about her weight constantly, no one is allowed to talk about it except other "big women." She will accept no nutritional advice because she knows everything there is to know about her condition.

What it comes down to is the following excuse: "I've always been this way. This is just how I am." If it weren't for the fact that she has developed type 2 diabetes, she wouldn't be seeing a doctor.

The other person I have in mind is Sean, also forty, an easygoing man who has worked his way up into management with a big construction company. Because he's over six foot four and spends too much time sitting at the office or watching TV at home, Sean has back problems. Recently I noticed that he looked 20 pounds thinner than the last time we met. I asked him what he did to lose the weight. He shrugged.

"I had to," he said. "The wife, she doesn't like me being fat."

But what did he actually do?

"I get bored sometimes and start snacking on chips and stuff in the evening, whatever's lying around. That's where I get my gut from. So I stopped." He smiled. "And the wife's happier now."

Between these two people is a stark contrast—one lost weight simply by being aware of where the problem came from and then changing it. Luckily, there was no serious compulsion or craving behind Sean's overeating. Cheryl, however, is conditioned to eat compulsively. She even describes herself as addicted to food; she likes having a disorder more than facing what it takes to overcome it. For her, eating is "just who I am." Sadly, fighting against her weight and losing the battle is also who she is.

Reality is whatever we perceive it to be. That's how reality, in all its vastness, become personal. In your personal reality, if you perceive your body as ugly, it will never be your ally. If you perceive weight loss as basically "too hard," it will stay that way. Ultimately, society has imposed secondhand beliefs that we perceive to be true. At best, they are somebody else's truths. Most of the time, they are just bricks used to build thicker walls around the prison.

Awareness Brings Freedom

For someone who has identified with being fat, the whole story has to change starting at a deep level. (A tiny minority among the obese declare that "fat is beautiful," and if they are proud to march to a different drummer, that's fine. Being proud won't reduce their serious health risks, however, and one generally notices a good deal of defensiveness in their attitude, which suggests that deeper, more negative feelings are present.) Such a person is literally a prisoner who has so little hope that they've learned to call prison their home. A mountain of negative experiences, memories, habits, failure, and frustration must be moved. The very thing they have given up on—freedom— needs to become the theme they follow and reinforce every day.

Fortunately, each of us is more than our brain. If you have a pizza in front of you and your brain has triggered the message "You must eat this" or even "You have to eat the whole thing," you can say no. People who can't say no feel like prisoners because their impulses have the upper hand. A part of them watches in dismay as the pizza gets eaten down to the last slice, like a helpless bystander watching a car crash in slow motion. But what is missing is actually basic and simple: a window of freedom.

I'm talking about the small space that opens in your mind before you make a decision. When you eat normally, you are free to choose. You don't see a pizza and automatically react the way you were conditioned to react. Instead, there's a space between hunger and choice. In that space you ask yourself, "Am I hungry? How much do I want to eat? Is this the food I would ideally choose?" Someone who is compelled to eat the whole thing no longer enjoys freedom of choice.

The space between hunger and eating, where you make the choice you want to make, isn't empty. It is filled with awareness. Awareness is close to what people call an open mind. You are free to think the thoughts you want to have. Conditioning is the opposite of an open mind. You have no conscious control over your behavior—your brain is in charge, falling back into old, deep grooves created in the past.

The joy of awareness is that you can escape any limitation imposed on you. Don't try to find out where these limitations came from. The point is that your brain has accepted them. So the first step is to open a space where you—the user of the brain—can say no to the old pathways and start to build new ones.

Action Step:
New Thoughts for Old

When your brain is conditioned, it automatically sends the same thoughts to you over and over. Unless you step in with a new thought, the old pathways get reinforced. It's not hard to step in. You just have to make it a priority, backed up with a commitment to be free. Consider this a kind of replacement therapy.

Here are some typical thoughts dictated by poor body image, frustration, and bad habits. If you have such thoughts, stop and replace them as soon as they occur. Repeat the replacement thought several times until it sinks in. If the new thought feels uncomfortable or raises certain emotions, sit quietly with your eyes shut and let the reaction pass. Don't fight it. Just observe what's going on. When you feel centered again, repeat the new thought one more time.

Old thought: I did this to myself. It's all my fault.
New thought: Who cares whose fault it is? Assigning blame does no good—I want to focus all my energies on the solution.

Old thought: I'm weak and ugly. I'm not good enough.
New thought: I am good enough; I don't need to compare myself to others; it's not about good or bad. Even movie stars gain weight, so it's not about ugly.

Old thought: I'm a loser. Look at how many times I've failed.
New thought: In the past I didn't know what I know now. In the long run, dieting was never the right tactic. I'm going to change my story to one of fulfillment. If I'm not perfect at it, that's okay. I'm on a learning curve.

Old thought: I'm just kidding myself. Look at me. Nothing will ever work.
New thought: I don't need to keep looking at my body. I can look at my new story and how it is succeeding. My body will follow. Right now, I will find something I enjoy more than feeling sorry for myself.

Old thought: I don't have the time or energy to try to lose weight.

New thought: To be honest, I think about my weight all the time, so if I stop obsessing, I have plenty of time to change my story. I have plenty of energy to do what I really like, and right now, changing my story is something I really like.

Notice that you aren't simply taking negativity and changing it to positivity. That can work for a while, but at a certain point you lose motivation—negativity is triggered every time you look in the mirror or watch other people do things you can't do. This action step is about *giving your brain reasons to change*. The higher brain is in charge of rational choices and behavior. If you keep feeding it with new thoughts that contain rational solutions, these new thoughts will start to become imprinted as "my way of doing things." It's all part of changing your perception so that reality—meaning your personal reality—will change at the same time.

Conscious Versus Unconscious

Your whole lifestyle is shaped by how conscious you are. Every choice traces back to the mind. Many problems are rooted in the blanking out, denial, numbness, and conditioning that we've been discussing in this chapter. What lies ahead is a brighter vision, and in this vision you are leading a conscious life. It takes a conscious lifestyle to get there, and I've been showing you how to lead one, where your higher brain is freed from lower-brain impulses, drives, and cravings.

If you stand back from your present lifestyle, with all its positive and negative aspects, you will see that the appeal of being unconscious is strong—people wouldn't go into denial and run after distractions if it wasn't. At the same time, the appeal of being conscious is also real, even though society doesn't teach us that this is true. Mass advertising, not just for junk food but for every kind of consumer good, tries to make impulsiveness look exciting. The answer to everything is to consume more and more, as if masking pain with pleasure is the right solution.

It's really helpful to look at reality, showing what actually happens if you adopt a conscious lifestyle versus an unconscious one.

Unconscious Lifestyle

When you are unconscious, your life story isn't under your control. You're a brain puppet, which means that your choices aren't really your own. They are mechanical repetitions of past choices. You give in to momentary impulses. You make hasty decisions and regret them later. Unintended consequences seem to rise out of the ground like weeds. People who lead an unconscious lifestyle can't realistically solve their problems. They are prone to the following thoughts:

Why is this happening to me?
Why can't I get anything done?
Why do I feel so overwhelmed?
Somebody has to help me.
I'm out of control.

These are not pleasant thoughts, and they can easily lead to panic. Yet we all go unconscious under certain circumstances. In the face of heavy stress, we shut down from sheer exhaustion. Unable to solve a difficult personal issue, we resign ourselves to it. A mind-body process is at work, the natural instinct to avoid pain. An unconscious lifestyle detaches you from tough situations. In the short run this feels like a relief—your sensitivity to pain is lessened.

But in the long run, being unconscious involves too much avoidance. The negativity you are trying to shut out isn't resolved. Bad things continue to happen, and they increase, because when you don't develop good coping skills, you can't solve your problems. If you have gotten in the habit of being unconscious, you will procrastinate and keep putting off important decisions. You are likely to be forgetful and indecisive. It will be hard to speak your truth because you aren't really sure who you are.

Typical Feelings from Being Unconscious

Impulsiveness
Depression
Anxiety
Restlessness
Victimization
Helplessness

Being Conscious

When you are conscious, you have control over your impulses. Your brain hasn't turned you into its puppet. Instead, you use the brain as the mind's magnificent gift. It turns your intentions into reality, makes dreams come true, and delivers a stream of creativity. The higher brain is mined for its resources of intelligence and evolution. When you lead a conscious lifestyle, you can make rational decisions, which gives you the power to shape your future. Unforeseen consequences are much less, and when they arise, you trust that you can find a solution. You are not fortune's fool.

To be conscious is to know how to deal with unpredictability and uncertainty. Experience has taught you that uncertainty has its own wisdom—without it, life would be boringly predictable. So surf the wave of uncertainty; instead of going under, be alert and responsive to the changing situations in your life. When you lead a conscious lifestyle, a snapshot of your mind would include thoughts like the following:

I need to plan ahead.
I'm in control.
What's my best choice in this situation?
Are things working out the way they should?
Let me think about this for a while. I need time to consider.
I know what I'm doing.

These are considered thoughts that bring reassurance. The more conscious you are, the more you feel in charge—you are writing a proud, satisfying story. No one is writing it for you, and if they try, you will go to considerable lengths to reclaim your rights. Consciousness is also associated with mastering a skill. Mastery requires the ability to remember and learn from our mistakes, to have patience with the learning curve, and to postpone immediate results for long-term gains. Consciousness opens the way for success in meeting life's challenges.

Typical Feelings from Being Conscious

Awakeness
Alertness
Interest
Curiosity
A Settled Feeling
Assuredness
Openness
Flexibility

One reason we've been focusing on themes is that unlike simple advice, a theme is something you can take hold of and be creative with. Bringing any of them into your life—whether it's lightness, purity, energy, or balance—brings you out of an unconscious lifestyle into a conscious one. Getting to our ideal weight is important, but to be honest, scanning the many books on diet, nutrition, and weight control, even the most reliable (which are in a slim minority) don't change a person's life as much as they promise to. Only awareness can do that.

When you achieve a conscious lifestyle, you will celebrate your whole existence. Keep that in mind every day. Make it your vision, and shape all your choices around it. Here's a version of my own personal vision. It's a manifesto, which grew out of the right to be aware. Adopt it; personalize it. When you feel that you've lost focus, take out your manifesto and reinforce it as much as you can.

A Mindful Manifesto

I expect my body to project what I want.
I want to be at my ideal weight.
I want to feel light, energetic, and joyful.
I want to be pain free.
I want to feel good about how my body looks.
I want to be rested and centered.
I want to be in a state of well-being.

Your old conditioning is preventing you from living your manifesto today in all its fulfillment. But nothing can stop you from having a vision, and once you pursue it, life expands its possibilities as your awareness expands. The world's wisdom traditions have made this promise for thousands of years, and countless people have found fulfillment on the path you are now walking.

Making It Personal:
"How Am I Doing?"

A ll actions begin in the mind, so learning to direct your mind is a prerequisite for any type of change. I find a lot of truth in the saying, "You are only as safe as your thoughts." If your thoughts are about temptation, not giving in, irresistible cravings, and being powerless to control your weight, you don't feel safe. How much you weigh isn't the key here. The key is staying in weight-loss awareness. We can break weight-loss awareness down into the following:

Not fighting against yourself

Ignoring calorie counting

Giving up diet foods

Eating natural foods

Knowing how hungry you are

Restoring balance where it matters

Dealing with things that bring you out of balance

Focusing on reaching your desired goal of ideal weight

Finding satisfaction without overeating

When someone is firmly in weight-loss awareness, they are walking the path—no matter what you do at the level of action, all paths are actually in awareness, the place where all beliefs, hopes, wishes, dreams, and fears get activated.

Today, take a few moments in the morning to review your state of mind. Rate yourself on each element of weight-loss awareness from 1 to 5:

5. I've got this down—I'm proud of where I am.

4. I'm doing okay.

3. I need to pay more attention.

2. I've slipped up—I need to really focus.

1. Uh-oh, I completely forgot this.

Take the item that you most want to change, and during your day make mental space to work on it. Your aim is to offer your brain a simple reminder. With repetition, this turns into a powerful tool for retraining your brain.

At the same time, take note of where you are succeeding. Appreciate how well you are doing. Really identify with your positive state of awareness—it's the thing that is going to change your life.

Self-Regulation

Let Your Body Take Care of You

Power Points

- Your body/mind is a self-regulating system. Self-regulation is called homeostasis—dynamic nonchange in the midst of change.
- All bodily functions are self-regulated through feedback loops. Your thoughts, feelings, and desires are the most important input your body receives in the loops.
- The signals for body awareness are satiety/hunger, comfort/discomfort, energy/lethargy, and lightness/heaviness.
- Hundreds of feedback loops function effortlessly to keep you alive, healthy, vital, and moving without your conscious participation. But your input is needed to maintain important biorhythms, especially sleep.
- Optimal biorhythms are related to optimal metabolism, which leads to more energy and normal weight. Impaired biorhythms create hormonal imbalances, disrupting many feedback loops. Overweight exacerbates the negative effects.
- Your body is aware of itself as a symphony of intermeshed processes. It doesn't see itself as a machine or a "thing." You should consider your body a verb, not a noun.

Y ou can ignore your body, but your body will never ignore you. It has faithfully taken care of you since the moment you were conceived. No matter how much you neglect or abuse it, your body doesn't abandon its mission. It exists to take care of you, if only you will let it. When you go unconscious at night during sleep, your body continues to regulate thousands of processes with no attention from you. Your body's mission is to keep you alive, healthy, and moving. This ability is known as self-regulation—fifty trillion cells operating on the honor system, so to speak.

If you consciously let your body take care of you, it will become your greatest ally and trusted partner. The most important thing you can do right now is to stop interfering with self-regulation. In cases of serious overweight, the interference takes physical form. Added weight puts unnecessary pressure on the whole system. If the body is like a supercomputer, constantly processing input and output, it wouldn't help to pour melted beef fat and caramel into a computer.

I say that only slightly tongue in cheek because the works get gummed up far worse when you throw in mental and emotional toxins. Every negative belief weakens the partnership between mind and body. We've lightly touched on a key issue known as homeostasis, the body's ability to preserve nonchange in the midst of activity. Those abstract words point to the miraculous abilities of self-regulation. Life is structured to keep self-regulation out of sight so that you can do what you want to do. You might put on your jogging clothes, thinking, "It's time to go around the park," which seems like a simple message. You are asking your body to get moving. But at a hidden level, your instruction affects blood sugar, cholesterol, blood pressure, body temperature, body fat, muscle mass, bone density, hormone levels, metabolic activity, immune function, and body weight. There's never a moment when every one of these functions isn't being regulated. And the main goal is homeostasis, letting you do something dynamic (jogging around the park) while maintaining a constant state of balance in your body.

If homeostasis gets thrown off, your body sends you a signal. For example, maybe you haven't jogged for three months and are suddenly inspired by a beautiful spring day to jog around the park. Unprepared for your sudden decision, your body does everything it can to take care of you. But pushed too far, it will send you signals of discomfort and strain: You feel winded, your muscles are weak, your joints ache, your breathing becomes ragged, you feel your heart pounding in your chest. These are the automatic results of homeostasis being pushed to the point where you must intervene. What you do next is up to you.

How Body Awareness Works

Too many processes are simultaneously going on in the human body to think of it as a noun. As I mentioned earlier, I like to think of the body as a verb. Your conscious mind can't possibly monitor all the biological processes in the body. The basic signals that your body wants you to be aware of embrace the themes that we've been working with:

Satiety/hunger
Comfort/discomfort
Energy/lethargy
Lightness/heaviness

The first term in each pair indicates a state of balance—homeostasis is taking care of you without undue pressure, stress, and strain. The second word in each pair indicates that homeostasis is under pressure. You are receiving feedback from an automatic system that needs you to consciously correct the situation. If you make the correction, self-regulation returns to its normal miraculous operation, and everything starts to hum again.

The best way to correct imbalance is through body awareness, which is basically effortless. You monitor how you feel, paying attention to the primary signals listed above: satiety/hunger, comfort/discomfort, energy/lethargy, and lightness/heaviness.

Action Step:
Awareness of Hunger

The more fine-tuned your awareness, the more in touch with your body you will be. Too often we say, "I'm famished" and reach for a lot of food when the body is actually saying, "I'm a little bit hungry" and would be satisfied with half a sandwich or a green salad.

The next time you're hungry, stop and rate your hunger on a scale from 0 to 8.

0 to 1 Your stomach is completely empty—you cannot feel the presence of food in your system from the previous meal. At the same time, there is a sensation of hunger. This is the point at which you should start eating.

2 to 4 This is how you feel when you are eating comfortably, or after you've just eaten and are comfortably digesting the food. You do not feel hunger at these levels.

5 As you are eating, you start to feel satisfied.

6 This is the point of maximum comfort. You feel completely satisfied—there is neither a sensation of hunger nor any discomfort from overeating. This is the level at which you should stop eating.

7 to 8 You have gone beyond the level of comfort. After eating there is a sensation of discomfort, such as heaviness, dullness, and distension of the abdomen.

Many people feel compelled to eat even when, according to their bodies, they are full already. They may not be compulsive eaters, but these people are under some sort of pressure, in need of some kind of comfort. Or sometimes life just happens; for instance, a client might unexpectedly call and ask to meet for an early dinner, so going to a restaurant becomes mandatory only a few hours after a filling lunch.

Whatever your situation, being aware of your hunger level, and then obeying it, keeps the feedback loop between mind and body strong. Some tips:

• Obey your hunger level. Don't eat if you're already full. Conversely, don't starve yourself when you're famished (which people do in the belief that going hungry means they're losing weight).
• Keep in touch with your hunger level as you eat. When you are nicely full, which is around a 6 on the scale from 0 to 8, stop eating. Get up from the table or have your plate cleared away.
• Learn to appreciate the feeling of mild hunger as a positive message from your body. Don't use it as an excuse to instantly grab some food.

Being aware of your body comes naturally. If something aches, for example, discomfort is an unpleasant signal, and you instinctively want it to go away. But the mind's response isn't always so simple. For many overweight people, negative beliefs have been in place for so long that they barely get noticed. Even so, you can spot them through the damaging thoughts they generate. What kind of mind-body partnership is going on if you have thoughts like the following?:

My body is ugly and inferior.
I'm stuck with this body. There's nothing I can do about it.
No matter how hard I try to lose weight, my body won't cooperate.
I'm so disappointed in my body.

It's just a matter of time before something inside really goes wrong. The best thing is to ignore how my body looks and feels.

Clearly the partnership is in trouble. In my experience, people with a history of weight issues are generally quite detached from the mind-body connection. They certainly aren't using it to their benefit.

Amanda, a patient who came to me, had developed type 2 diabetes at age fifty-five after carrying too much weight since she was a teenager. I was just one in a long string of doctors she was seeing, which is no surprise since diabetes has systemic effects. Her eye doctor told Amanda that her blurry vision was the result of retinal deterioration, which fortunately was mild so far. Other doctors were addressing her fatigue, mood swings, oversensitivity to medications, erratic blood sugar, and lower back pain (this last was not related to her diabetes).

Amanda is a stoic and forthright woman. She trudges from doctor to doctor determined to fix these symptoms. The first thing she told me was, "I consider myself a healer. I do body work but it's holistic. My clients tell me I've changed their lives."

"And you wonder why you can't change yours," I interjected. She nodded.

I asked Amanda what she was doing for herself, and she rattled off an impressive list. She went to a wide array of alternative therapists. She took supplements and was extremely concerned with avoiding processed foods. She did a cleanse once a month. All of these steps were proactive, but there was a catch.

"I like the things you're doing," I said. "But how do you feel?" To me, she looked worried and tense.

"I'm frazzled," Amanda admitted. "I hate all these doctor visits. I just want these problems to go away."

"I get the idea that all this worry has made you eat more," I said. She had gained 10 pounds in the two months since our last appointment. Amanda nodded, looking distressed. Her body told her she was in trouble, but her answer to added stress was more food. So her body was no longer in partnership with her, and she needed to change that. There was lots of melodrama, too, along with the medical concerns.

"You care about the whole situation," I pointed out. "But you are caring in a negative way. Your body has gone so far out of balance that it's sending up distress flares. You have to get your body's distress down, and when you do, your own distress will decrease. The two are intimately connected."

The right kind of caring aids the body in restoring homeostasis; healing cannot progress until this happens. Amanda could do a lot to give her body a chance to reset itself:

She could stop eating so much.
She could take up meditation.
She could take proactive steps to reduce her stress levels.
She could examine her negative beliefs.
She could feed the mind-body connection with the positive reinforcements of fulfillment.

Those are all forms of positive feedback. I also had an immediate suggestion. I asked Amanda to close her eyes and sit quietly for a moment. Then I guided her through the following meditation:

"In your mind's eye, visualize your body as healthy and balanced. Visualize it at your ideal weight. Feel the contentment this brings. Visualize yourself smiling, feeling pleased with your body. Say to yourself, 'This is the real me. I want to have the body I'm seeing. It's going to be my body as soon as possible.'"

As she went through the meditation, Amanda smiled. You could see the tension flowing out of her system. Her face relaxed into a look of contentment and hope.

Why didn't Amanda's previous doctors help her? Because they looked on her body basically as a broken machine that needed to be fixed. They had little expertise—or interest—in the whole human picture. But the whole picture was of utmost importance to her. "Stop eating so much" was just the opening wedge of a mind-body strategy to get her into a better place in her life.

The Need for Feedback

Your body wants positive input. Its feedback loops work automatically, which is why you could survive in a coma for months or years. But the nervous system has a second half—the voluntary nervous system—that calls for your participation. It responds to what you say, think, and do.

Detachment means that you refuse to participate. You are instructing your brain and nervous system to carry on without you. That may sound neutral, but it isn't. Detachment takes various forms rooted in self-judgment. The main ones are denial, inertia, apathy, and resignation. People with weight issues know them all too well. Theirs is not the wise, calm detachment of a Buddha. Spiritual detachment is a state of peace. The kind of detachment that ignores what your body is telling you is born of negativity—there's nothing peaceful about it. A mix of toxic feelings and beliefs boils down to this: *My body is against me.*

It's important to turn that attitude around, because your body knows what you're thinking and feeling. You are feeding it your negativity. Trillions of cells are receiving chemical messages from your brain at every moment, encoded as chemicals. A stress hormone like cortisol plays a vital role in two functions essential to life: eating and sleeping. When I studied it as an endocrinologist, our whole focus was on the structure of the cortisol molecule and how it interacted with other hormones. The interaction was complex and fascinating. I was mesmerized by how a sudden stress, like hearing the words "You're fired," instantly causes a spurt of stress hormones, and two minutes later, the entire body has changed—all from two words.

Now I use that clue to see cortisol not as a molecule but primarily as a threat. "You're fired" is being sent through the bloodstream like a text message bringing bad news. We ignored the messages in medical training because everything was materialistic; the human side was secondary. But of course "You're fired" is a human message, and so are the negative thoughts about being overweight. "You're fat" are two words that no one wants to hear, and they can be just as devastating as, or perhaps more devastating than, "You're fired."

Hormones Reset Your Body

Let's look more closely at what you body is doing with the messages that constantly circulate through it. There are hundreds of feedback loops, and being interconnected, they regulate each other. So how can you reset them in a simple, effective way?

As I've already mentioned, the most important factor in homeostasis is balance, but in physiological terms, what is being balanced, exactly? The key elements are daily cycles known as biorhythms. Bodily processes aren't random. They are rhythmic, and each rhythm is meshed with every other, like an imaginary clock shop where a hundred clocks keep the same time even though they tick-tock at different rates. Your blood pressure, for example, follows a daily wave pattern as it goes up and down. The hormone cortisol tracks the rhythm of waking and sleeping (throwing this chemical cycle off leads to the bad effects of jet lag or working the night shift—although night workers may think they have adjusted to being awake when they should be asleep, their cortisol levels tell a different story).

The menstrual cycle in women depends on hormones, and although the causes of premenstrual syndrome (PMS) aren't well understood, researchers have suspected that a cyclical shift in hormones, accompanied by changes in the brain, may be key. With a different physiology, men are hormonal, too, and if you do a Google search for "male period," you will find advocates of a male monthly cycle of testosterone, linked to moodiness, sexual arousal, and depression. Medically, such a cycle has been little reported and less studied, but testosterone does go through a daily cycle, peaking in the morning.

There's a symphony of hormones coursing through your body, and when they are balanced with one another, your biorhythms follow a natural pattern. When your body is out of balance, hormone levels reflect that, too. Lack of sleep, for example, as it throws off your cortisol levels, affects the hunger response, which is why people tend to eat more when their sleep is bad. This factor is so important that losing your natural sleep rhythm could be the key to why you overeat (for people with chronic depression, the first sign of an attack can be irregular sleep, and if this is attended to immediately, the oncoming depression may not arrive).

Hormones are regulators, or gatekeepers. They keep the most important bodily functions within a certain range, neither too high nor too low. This includes breathing, drinking water, eating food, digestion, metabolism, elimination of waste, and sensory experience through sound, touch, sight, taste, and smell. All must be self-regulated within the right limits. If you are suddenly frightened and your breathing becomes fast and ragged (a physical sign of fight-or-flight), a hormone—adrenaline—has pushed your heart to its upper extreme. Your body knows that this extreme can be safely maintained only for a short while, so adrenaline passes quickly from the system.

How are hormones relevant to being overweight? We've already discussed how eating too much or eating the wrong foods throws off your blood sugar, affecting insulin levels and posing a risk for developing diabetes (although being prediabetic is also unhealthy; you aren't safe just because disease symptoms haven't appeared yet). More troubling perhaps is belly fat that develops around the waist. Just the fact that the fat is placed here on your body makes a difference. Women before the onset of menopause who carry abdominal fat were seen to have inferior bone quality and lower bone formation than women who carried their fat elsewhere on their bodies.

In both sexes, the adverse effect of belly fat, which has only recently been targeted by researchers, is that these fat cells constantly secrete hormones into the bloodstream. In particular, they introduce leptin, the hormone that increases your appetite, which is naturally counterbalanced by ghrelin, the hormone for satiety. It's been found that leptin levels are directly proportional to body weight. In other words, the more you weigh, the hungrier you'll feel, which is a cruel irony, since of course body fat is nature's backup for when food becomes scarce. Leptin is also central in metabolizing fat, and this too is cyclical. Your fat metabolism is highest 9 to 10 hours after you eat dinner at night. Introducing a snack before you go to bed is thought to interfere with the cycle. You are causing trouble in two ways, by taking in food when the body doesn't want it and by inhibiting its ability to metabolize fat.

Leptin is also tied into the "diets don't work" syndrome. The rebound effect after people come off a crash diet and regain the pounds they lost, with a few more added on, is related to increased leptin. Your body reads a crash diet as a famine, since both bring drastically fewer calories. When the famine is over, leptin levels rise to make you hungrier while at the same time your metabolism is adjusted—also by hormones—to turn more food into fat. The trick of eating a bit of food an hour before a meal works because it triggers the leptin/ghrelin cycle to move from eating to metabolism, when hunger is naturally suppressed.

Action Step:
Connecting Food, Mood, and Energy

Medical science validates how what you eat and how you feel are connected through a symphony of hormones. But you are the best judge of your own situation. Now that you have learned to use an appetite scale for your true hunger levels, it can be linked to how eating affects your mood and energy level.

For the next two weeks, keep a daily log that tracks these three factors—here's a template for how each page will look:

	Appetite Level Before Eating	Appetite Level After Eating	Mood Before Eating	Mood After Eating	Energy Level Before Eating	Energy Level After Eating
Breakfast						
Lunch						
Dinner						

To gauge your mood, use a scale of 1 to 10, where 10 is a state of blissful well-being and joy and 1 represents feelings of deep unhappiness or emotional pain. Also rate your energy levels on a scale of 1 to 10, with 10 indicating the highest level of vibrant energy, and 1 the feeling of being wiped out and too tired to get out of bed.

In my own experience keeping track of my appetite, mood, and energy levels, I began to notice patterns emerging. For example, when I stopped eating at levels 4 to 6 (associated with a light meal), I almost always felt energized and content. If I let myself get too full, however, I persistently noticed that I felt sluggish and uninspired.

In the opposite direction, if I waited too long to eat, letting myself dip to a 1 or 2 on the appetite gauge, I might wind up devouring the next meal, feeling tired, or getting irritable.

Keep in mind that the daily log is a mindfulness tool to help you increase self-awareness. Simply observe any patterns without judging or criticizing yourself. As your awareness expands, you will naturally be guided to make any shifts in your eating that help you feel happier and more energetic.

Stress Eating

Clearly your body needs to have normal hormone levels to stay in the flow of biorhythms. If biorhythms have gotten thrown off, you need to find a way to reset them. In terms of the imbalance caused by weight gain, it's useful to divide overweight people into two categories. The first category has issues with insulin and blood sugar. The main way to reset your body's insulin levels is through the foods you eat, concentrating on natural foods and avoiding refined sugar and other simple carbohydrates. I say more on this in the section on the Chopra Center's philosophy of food.

The second kind of overweight person has issues regarding stress. The connection between eating too much sugar and throwing your blood sugar out of balance is direct, but the link between stress and gaining weight is more indirect, involving some hormones that at first glance have little to do with hunger and body fat. Even so, they are woven into the symphony of hormones, because these chemicals do not act alone.

The dividing line between blood sugar issues and stress issues is vague, because no matter which category you fall into, once you gain extra body fat, those cells start secreting hormones that affect your blood sugar and appetite. Is this happening to you?

Quiz:
Are You a Stress Eater?

Check the items that apply to your eating and general situation.

____ Are you a woman? (Women are more likely to be stress eaters. They turn to food for comfort, whereas men are more likely to turn to alcohol and smoking.)

____ Are you sedentary, not engaging in regular exercise? (Exercise has the effect of making you hungry in the short term but seems to reset the stress response if you exercise vigorously on a regular basis.)

____ Are you lonely or isolated socially? (Lack of social support means that you don't have an outlet for releasing daily stresses.)

____ Do you snack when you are feeling nervous or restless?

____ Do you cope with stress entirely on your own?

____ Does daily stress and strain make it hard for you to fall asleep and keep sleeping for at least 7 to 8 hours? (Irregular sleep throws off the daily cortisol cycle.)

____ Do you find yourself grabbing food between meals to relieve boredom or pressure at work?

____ If you feel stressed, do you immediately reach for sugary, fatty snack foods?

Score: _____

Rating Yourself
If you checked *1 or 2 items,* you are likely not a stress eater. You haven't set up a feedback loop between daily stress and food. A score of *5 to 8 items* puts you firmly in the category of stress eating. You are coping with life using food, and a feedback loop has been set up so that the more you use food for comfort, the less effective it is, leading to even more eating.

What Should I Do?

Dealing with stress in a better way is the key to breaking the cycle of stress eating. Don't fight your appetite; teach your brain that you can cope with the stress response more effectively. As noted in the quiz, dealing with stress should include selections from the anti-stress menu:

Meditation
Yoga
Relaxation techniques, including breathing exercises
Good sleep
Exercise, if vigorous and regular
Close social connections

Stress is such a major suspect in America's obesity problems that it deserves detailed attention, so look at the "Making It Personal" section at the end of this chapter, which says a lot more about this issue, which affects most people in hidden ways even when they think they aren't leading a stressed-out life.

Stress eating is a paradox. In the short run, adrenaline, which triggers the fight-or-flight syndrome, shuts down the digestive tract and dampens your appetite. "I'm too upset to eat anything" is a first response to stress. (This is chemically linked to a gland in the brain, the hypothalamus, which secretes corticotropin-releasing hormone, which essentially says to the body, "This is an emergency. It's no time to eat.") Some people are nervous eaters, and they remain thin; being overreactive to small, everyday stresses, their hormones keep them from feeling hungry.

But in the aftermath of stress, thanks to the hormone cortisol, which stokes appetite and provides strong motivation, you can find yourself driven to eat. After fighting a battle or winning a football game, a person is so charged up that eating becomes a big, immediate need. Cortisol levels naturally fall after a stress has passed, but if the stress is constant, even though it's low-level, eating can become compulsive. (I remember the touching story of a man who had just lost his wife, and as part of his grieving, he found himself driving all night down the Pacific Coast Highway, stopping at every roadside diner to have a steak.)

Although the research here is less clear, stress seems to make people crave sugary and fatty foods. It is thought that this is another hormone-controlled feedback loop, because sugar and fat seem to suppress the part of the brain that responds to stress. There's a physiological reason a big piece of chocolate cake is comfort food. The secret isn't to keep eating more and more chocolate cake to remain comforted—that leads to disaster as far as your body is concerned—but to deal with the stress that has thrown off your hormone balance.

Thirty-five years ago, when I was in training and first became interested in what were then dubbed "molecules of emotion," an amazing landscape opened up. Hormones are the key to self-regulation, and the mind-body connection was impossible to ignore once you saw how dramatically hormones are involved in how we think, how we feel, how we behave—and how we eat. Earlier we looked into the four hormones directly connected to eating (leptin, ghrelin, insulin, and adiponectin). Although they don't take center stage, four other hormones are at play in weight issues:

Adrenaline
Cortisol
Endorphins
Thyroid hormones

The two stress hormones, adrenaline and cortisol, were never linked to weight until it was discovered that they increase deposits of belly fat. Endorphins, the natural opiates manufactured in the brain, function as painkillers. They increase with exercise, falling in love, having an orgasm, and eating spicy foods. There's no single message there, until you stand back and realize that endorphins are one ingredient in the body's "satisfaction cocktail." As such, their rise and fall clearly meshes with the whole picture of how fulfilled you are and what you do to find more fulfillment.

I'm not asking you to memorize the functions of every hormone—exactly the opposite. Your hormones are orchestrated and intertwined. They translate your feelings into chemical messages that your cells can understand. It's amazing that this can happen, and no one knows how it really works. Why should a chemical, adrenaline, make you have the feeling of fear or the desire to run away? Science cannot say, but the crucial point is that hormones allow you to maintain a state of inner balance and peace while also giving you the possibility of quick response to any change in your life.

What this means for your weight is that you must look beyond a single "hunger hormone" or "fat hormone" to take in the whole picture. The textbook description of hormones is too narrow, being totally disconnected from the human situation. The thyroid always comes up in any discussion on metabolism and obesity. To an endocrinologist the connection among thyroid activity, emotions, and metabolism is not clear-cut. But it makes sense that a low thyroid level linked to depression or stress will influence your metabolism. That's a simple example of looking at the whole picture, considering why someone in a negative emotional state will be sending hormonal signals to the body that have a widespread effect. (In the chapter on emotional well-being, three more hormones are added to the chemical symphony.)

Sleep, the Master Biorhythm

Hormones give us a label for how totally interconnected the mind and body are. Change one important biorhythm, and the effects will be felt everywhere. This is most important with sleep, which is the master biorhythm that sets everything else for the day. As you probably know, the reason we sleep remains a mystery. Almost all the discoveries made in sleep research come from sleep deprivation. Force someone to stay awake, and shortly the first symptoms—dullness, decreased coordination, mental fog, and physical fatigue—appear. If a person is forced to stay awake beyond twenty-four hours, which is hard to induce even in the laboratory, symptoms become severe, leading to hallucinations and chaotic physical processes in the body.

Because sleep research is conducted through deprivation, we find ourselves in much the same position as the study of vitamins, which is done through vitamin deficiencies. Taking away vitamin C leads to scurvy, among other disorders, but this doesn't tell you how to optimize vitamin C, which is the other half of the story, and certainly the more important half for everyday life.

As far as sleep goes, the sad truth is that we have to begin with deprivation, given that half of American adults report problems getting a good night's sleep during the past week, and two-thirds say that they should be getting more sleep. What defeats good sleep? To begin with:

- Taking work home with you
- Anxiety
- Eating late at night
- Too much noise or light in the bedroom
- Jet lag
- Illness
- Minor aches and pains

- Certain medications
- Interruptions to urinate
- Irregular habits
- A history of insomnia
- Accumulated stress

All of these factors can easily be connected to overeating. But just by itself, lack of sleep throws off hormone balance, and one result is that you get hungry and also can't control what you eat (because your decision-making ability is decreased). Leptin, ghrelin, and cortisol are thrown off their normal rhythms. There are secondary effects, too. Lack of sleep can make you irritable or depressed, and this in turns leads you to eat in order to feel better.

It may be scientifically valid that some people are programmed to be night owls, not feeling sleepy until after midnight and needing to sleep in late, while others are programmed to go to bed early and wake up early. Anyone who has lived with someone who falls into the opposite category knows firsthand how hard this programming is to change. No real research has been done to verify whether change is even possible with such a basic biorhythm.

But two things are beyond dispute. Sleep is cyclical. Sleep is chemical. Because it's cyclical, you should do your best to respect your body's attunement to the rhythm of the seasons and the changes from light to dark. Because sleep is chemical, realize that your brain must secrete certain substances to get you to sleep and wake you up again. Interfering with these chemicals by using alcohol, tobacco, or drugs is a major don't. But even to throw your sleep time off by wide variances in your routine is like volunteering for jet lag or the night shift, two things that sleep doesn't like.

The guidelines for getting a good night's sleep are well known and should be tried before you consider whether you have anything close to a sleep disorder.

What Leads to Sound Sleep?

1. Observe routine hours for going to bed.

2. Have the bedroom as dark as possible. Even low light levels activate the pineal gland, a small region in the brain that regulates daily rhythms according to light and dark.

3. Have the room as quiet as possible. As you sleep, you rise into periods that are almost awake, and even minor sounds (a ticking clock or dripping bathroom faucet) can wake you up prematurely.

4. Set the temperature on the cool side, since your body warms up in bed, and too much warmth may wake you up.

5. Eliminate minor aches and pains. These become more noticeable when you go to bed. Half an aspirin before bedtime may be all you need.

6. Don't be mentally active for an hour before going to bed.

7. Don't go to bed angry or upset.

8. Resist tossing and turning. Lie still and wait for sleep to come naturally.

9. Arrange your bedtime so that you get a comfortable 8 hours of uninterrupted sleep.

10. If you are prone to getting up to urinate, don't drink liquids for 2 hours before going to bed.

11. Wake up without an alarm, allowing the natural wake-sleep cycle to reset itself.

If you have tried all of these measures—not once but for at least two weeks—and you still have problems getting to sleep, a multitude of advice can be found on the Internet. Yet current research seems somewhat contradictory. It used to be thought that if you didn't get a good night's sleep during the workweek, you couldn't make up for it by sleeping in on the weekend. It was also thought that the stages of deep sleep and REM sleep (REM stands for rapid eye movements, observed when someone is dreaming) were achieved only in 7 to 8 hours of uninterrupted sleep.

Now it seems that deep sleep and REM can be reached much more quickly, so researchers support the value of taking a catnap and catching up with extra hours of sleep if there is a deficit. But I'd make the point that sleep research can't be separated from the whole business of living. Nothing interrupts sleep worse than grief, stress, loss, failure, anxiety, depression, and everyday worries. In bad cases of insomnia, you must often look to other areas of your life. That's what we've been doing with eating and awareness; sleeping and awareness call for the same perspective. Most of the same answers also apply:

You will sleep well if you are happy.

The more contented you are, the better you will sleep.

Too much inertia and stagnation hurt your sleep; being active and engaged helps your sleep.

Being sluggish and tired leads to bad sleep, and in turn bad sleep makes you more sluggish and tired.

Toxins and reliance on medications, including sleep aids, throw off biorhythms and often cause sleep problems.

I'm not saying that when you go through a spell of insomnia, you need to look at your whole life. Be familiar with stress—covered in the "Making It Personal" section that follows—and become more aware of what is throwing your body off. Taking proactive steps is much better than turning into a victim and thrashing around randomly for quick fixes.

A small survey that friends and I came up with includes some sleep aids that are harmless—and at least one person swears by each of them:

- During the first 5 minutes in bed, review your day. See every significant event. Feel good about your day, and whatever remains undone or not well finished, know that you can handle it tomorrow. This exercise eases the state of low-level worry and substitutes a sense of satisfaction—nothing is more valuable.

- Lie on your back and keep your eyes open. If they start to close, focus on keeping them open. This trick works because it is the opposite of "trying to fall asleep," which is impossible.
- Lie perfectly still on your back. Your muscles are paralyzed during deep sleep, and by imitating this immobility, your brain is triggered to enter the sleep state.
- See the number 100 in your mind's eye. If the image fades or your mind wanders, go back to seeing the number. The trick here is that people are often kept awake by their thoughts. Seeing an image isn't cognitive—there are no words or thoughts. Therefore, by focusing on the number 100, you stop thinking about things too much.

Making It Personal: Dealing with Stress, without Eating

If you want to break the habit of eating when you feel stressed, you need a better way to handle stress. It's helpful to first learn a bit more about stress itself, especially the so-called normal stress of daily life. It's considered normal for two reasons. No traumatic event triggers the stress, and the kind of pressure we all feel is generally low-level. It tends to fly beneath the radar. But if you find yourself eating without being able to put your finger on why you suddenly wanted food, it's likely that you are trying to cope with stress.

Food, even though comforting, shouldn't be your main way to cope, and certainly not the first one you reach for. Three factors make stress worse in daily life (see page 174).

Ineffectual Coping

How many of the following behaviors do you fall into when you find yourself feeling stressed?:

___I reach for food if I feel stressed.

___I react emotionally and sometimes blow up.

___I feel panicky and suffocated. I have to shut the stress out or run away.

___I ignore the stress and look for a distraction like watching TV, going online, or playing a video game.

___I complain about the pressure I'm under, mostly to people who aren't causing it.

___I pass the stress down the line, unloading it on someone else.

___I turn my back on the people who cause me the most stress, blocking them out as much as I can.

___I put up with stress until I get a chance to unwind hours later (e.g., going to the gym, having a cocktail).

___I create even more pressure on myself and others, on the theory that it makes me stronger and more competitive.

These behaviors don't achieve what they set out to do—decrease the harmful effects of stress. Stress is a feedback loop. The input is the stressor (e.g., a tight deadline, an obnoxious boss, an unreachable sales goal); the output is your response. You have a choice to intervene anywhere along the loop. The more consciously you intervene, the higher your chances of reducing the bad effects of stress.

Having seen what doesn't work, what does?

- Being aware of what's happening around you
- Monitoring how you feel inside
- Not stuffing down your emotions
- Finding ways to gain control over your life
- Insisting on lower stress where you can
- Knowing more about the mechanics of stress

Thanks to self-regulation, your body returns to balance after a stress occurs. You might jump because you hear a car backfire close by, but a few minutes later there will be no hint that your heart beat faster and your blood pressure rose. However, three factors can mount over time to prevent rebalancing, pushing you gradually into chronic imbalance:

Repetition

Unpredictability

Lack of control

Look upon these as the Big Three when it comes to chronic stress, because they can make the difference, literally, between life and death. In one classic laboratory experiment in animal behavior, mice were placed on a metal grid that administered a mild shock, not enough to harm them but enough to jolt them. The shocks were administered at random, and the mice could not run away. Thus the three worst factors—repetition, unpredictability, and lack of control—were all present.

Even though the shocks, considered one at a time, were harmless, the mice quickly declined and died. Their bodies' ability to return to homeostasis had been exhausted. Unable to adapt, they shut down completely. The lesson seems clear: Low-level stress appears to be harmless, but under the wrong conditions it leads to a breakdown of your ability to adapt.

If you want to deal with stress consciously, break it down into the following three components and minimize them in your feedback loop.

Repetition: Doing the same thing over and over dulls the mind; in and of itself, this is stressful, because shutdown is taking place. Exposed to any repetitive stress (e.g., doing cold calls as a salesman, dealing with the same incompetent employee, putting up with a boss's boorish behavior), the brain seeks a way to cope, falling back on a familiar pattern. Depending on your temperament, you will find yourself reacting with anger, frustration, suppressed resentment, boredom, or putting up a mental block—the tactic of stonewalling. These coping mechanisms cease to work over time, and then it takes smaller stresses to create a negative reaction.

Once you recognize a repetitive stress, you face other choices. If you find the repetition intolerable (for example, if there's the same loud noise over and over), walk away. If you are only a bit dulled by repetition, add a little spice and variety to your routine (e.g., instead of listening to the same boring people at work, talk to someone new). Most people are somewhere in between. They can't walk away or change the situation without making waves. In that case, you have to work on yourself. It helps to identify all the nagging, repetitive things that irritate you and change your routine to eliminate or at least ease them. As you take note of what these repetitive stresses are, for each one be aware of how you are presently coping. Ask yourself if there's a better way, and then adopt it.

Unpredictability: This kind of stress is perhaps worse than repetitive stress, because when you can't predict the next bad thing, you remain vigilant and apprehensive even when it's not happening. Children from homes where there is domestic abuse grow up to be hypervigilant. They cannot accept a normal state of calm when things are going well because they are conditioned to see this as merely the calm before the storm. There is always another shoe to drop.

If you find yourself looking over your shoulder in anticipation of something bad, or if you dwell on worst-case scenarios, your enemy is unpredictability. If the stress is coming from an emotionally unpredictable person, stay away. Your chances of changing their mood swings, outbursts of rage, or wayward job performance are slim to none. If the unpredictability comes from external forces, do what you can to make them more predictable or organize a coping strategy (parents of infants are doing this when they take turns each night getting out of bed to handle the crying baby). Opening yourself to feelings of anxiety and apprehension is the worst thing you can do. Arm yourself with scenarios that reasonably fit the next turn of events, without letting your imagination run away with you; then you will be reducing their unpredictability. That's how firefighters and police officers are trained to deal with many kinds of situations, so that they don't have to improvise at the scene.

Lack of control: I'd count this as the worst factor in stress. Having control over your life is important; it's probably the main reason that people start their own business or, more and more often, choose to live alone. Controlling personality types go further, trying to manage every detail of their lives, not to mention the people around them. Yet for anyone, lack of control creates frustration and a sense of helplessness. It does no good to simply become passive, since bottled-up frustration presents its own set of problems.

The best remedy is to assert control where it counts. You can't tell your boss where to go, and you can't turn your back on your workload, either. Instead, assert yourself where control is possible, for instance:

Insist on respect from others.

Ask for a dignified work environment.

Give other people their own space and ask for the same in return.

Work on things that you do best.

Take on a workload that isn't overburdening you.

Ask for monetary rewards commensurate with what you accomplish.

Insist on a minimum of busywork.

Don't be held to perfectionist standards.

Receive criticism, if you must, in private.

Insist on never being attacked personally.

Make alliances that can be trusted, without the risk of betrayal.

Ask to be valued for your knowledge and experience.

The wording of this list focuses on the workplace, although the same values apply at home and with your friends. As you look over each item, consider whether you have let things slide to the point of being stressful. If so, take corrective action. You deserve to write your own story, and being in control is an important element of any story.

We should talk a little more about stress at work. Modern work, like modern life in general, is set up to undermine the individual's sense of being in control. With huge forces amassed against you, from the demand for corporate profits to the undercutting of job and pension security, the need for you to assert control becomes greater. This isn't control for its own sake, or to show who is top dog. This is control as a means of reducing everyday pressures. When you can accomplish that, you open the field for a much more conscious approach to your life. On the other hand, if you deal with pressure unconsciously, your awareness will become constricted, and then the possibilities for your future narrow down at the same time.

So far we've covered the stress that affects you, but there are also times when you might be adding to the stress of others. It's good to focus some attention on relieving the stress you may be causing. A conscious person takes responsibility for both. Just remember that stress is a feedback loop, and the more you can do to improve your input, the more benefit you will receive in return.

You are creating unnecessary stress in the lives of others if you indulge in the following behaviors:

You are demanding, critical, and perfectionist—the perfect recipe for stress.

You give erratic orders and are prone to unpredictable changes.

You show disrespect for other workers and/or their work.

You create an undignified work environment (e.g., a place where swearing, gossip, and sexual remarks are commonplace).

You don't give other people their own space.

You pass your own workload to others just because you can.

You burden others with personal issues you should deal with yourself.

You criticize a subordinate in public.

You make personal attacks.

You can't be trusted.

You indulge in casual betrayals.

You devalue another worker's experience and knowledge.

These are more than bad behaviors. They trigger the stress response in other people, which is easily recognized, because they would trigger the same in you if you were on the receiving end. It's a myth that a hard-boiled attitude, confrontational tactics, and constant pressure are good for productivity. The best workplaces give people space, encourage creativity, allow workers to define their own work hours, assign tasks according to a worker's strengths, and create an atmosphere of general respect.

The signs of stress may be subtle, but when you pay attention, they are unmistakable. Let's say that you could possibly be stressing someone else out, once again focusing on work, knowing that the same signs may exist at home. People don't look happy being under you. They avoid direct eye contact. They miss work or shirk during work hours. They seem nervous in your presence. The atmosphere grows quiet and tense when you enter a room or give orders. There is silent resistance to giving you what you ask for—you have to ask a second time, and even then there are delays. People under you make excuses, or else they have lost their motivation to perform. (Substitute *your children* or *your spouse* in place of *people under you,* and you can see how much of this applies to home life as well.) If you don't identify with being in charge, maybe there's someone in your life who makes you act in these ways.

All of these symptoms are obvious. It doesn't matter if you are the CEO of a multinational corporation or a father sitting at the head of the dinner table. Stress is a threat in any situation, which is why we need to devote the next chapter to the opposite of stress, the desirable goal of emotional well-being.

Emotional Well-Being

It's a Choice

Power Points

- When you are more aware, you can make better choices. These choices either add to your sense of emotional well-being or detract from it.
- Like your body, your mind sends signals about its overall state. The signals for mental awareness are joy/suffering, love/fear, compassion/selfishness, peace (equanimity)/lack of peace.
- A basic key to happiness is to make each day happy.
- People who report that they are happy have a common trait: they actively connect with friends and loved ones for an hour or two a day.
- Yet there is no fixed program for ensuring happiness, because it cannot be quantified. Experiences of pleasure and pain, which can be quantified, aren't the same as well-being.
- In a state of restful alertness, the mind is balanced and open to the constant change that life brings.

W hen you bring awareness to any aspect of your life, you will reap benefits, because awareness tells you how you are doing. It's an infallible kind of radar, if you turn it on. Awareness allows you to sort out what you're doing, how you feel, what you fear, hope, and wish for—indeed everything in your life. It's tragic that so many Americans either turn their awareness off or focus it on unhappy states, such as anxiety and depression, which affect millions of people. Obesity is an unhappy state of mind just as much as an unhappy state of the body.

Awareness is turned off when you live under the following circumstances:

You act unconsciously, following habits and rote behavior.
You let others take charge of your life.
You feel victimized and emotionally trapped.
You isolate yourself and have no close connections with others.
You act passive and resigned in the face of things that make you unhappy.
You don't really know what you want.

The last point is so critical that this entire book is based on coming to a better understanding of it. You must know what you want. Otherwise, you wind up drifting. Or your life gets channeled in undesirable directions. As we've already established, too many people put food into their mouths when they are hungry for attention, appreciation, love, and affection. What they really want is being redirected.

The human mind is incredibly complex, but it delivers some basic states that loom over all the thoughts and feelings you have in a day, the way a marble mosaic delivers a picture rather than a jumble of tiny colored stones. The signals sent by the mind operate like the body's signals of comfort and discomfort. When you are mentally aware, the primary signals are the following:

Joy/Suffering
Love/Fear
Compassion/Selfishness
Peace (equanimity)/Lack of peace

On the left are the messages that lead to emotional well-being. On the right are messages that detract from well-being. You have a choice which side of the equation you want to live on. Finding well-being doesn't happen by itself.

The Best of All Habits: Self-Awareness

When you monitor the messages your mind is giving you, you are practicing self-awareness. Body awareness is also included, as it must be if your goal is to connect mind and body. Just as when you tune in to your body to receive its messages, self-awareness tunes in to your inner world. Once you get into the habit, it becomes second nature. At any moment of the day, you can ask yourself:

Am I joyful or suffering?
Do I feel love or fear?
Am I being compassionate or selfish?
Am I at peace or do I feel a lack of peace?

People's lives would be transformed if they asked themselves these basic questions—so why don't they? The answer isn't a secret. The habit of tuning in to the world of emotions poses obstacles for all of us. If I had you with me in person, right this minute, and said, "Check inside and tell me how you feel," experience tells me that all kinds of things might happen:

You might resist and refuse to look inside.

You might be too afraid of what you will see in yourself.

You might get a false message, based on what you think you should feel.

You might feel two things at once, not being sure which one is really true.

You might become emotional because of a flood of unexpected feelings or memories.

Psychologists put labels on the obstacles that keep us from being comfortable with what our minds want to tell us: denial, repression, neurosis, obsession, anxiety—the list is quite long. But if you practice self-awareness, you can penetrate the mental fog, even if it seems thick. To take just one mental pair, let's say you check in to see if you are experiencing love or fear. These are simple words, yet behind them lies a world of inner experience. If *love* simply meant romance and *fear* simply meant feeling terrified, most people wouldn't gain much when they tuned in. So let's apply more self-awareness and look at what love can be:

Knowing that there is mutual caring: you are both loved and loving

Enjoying what you're doing

Appreciating where you are

Feeling good about who you are

Having a loving, stable relationship

Feeling that your life is vibrant and stimulating

Experiencing a deep connection with a higher kind of love

If you pause for a moment and focus your awareness, you will know if you are experiencing these things, which make love more expansive and deeper. It's not just about feeling romantic. People who can give positive responses to each of these things worked to get there. They wrote a life story that included love, that found the courage to look into the opposite of love, which is fear, and then made choices that led out of fear.

Fear is also more than simply feeling afraid or terrified. Fear is about the following:

Feeling insecure
Not trusting what is happening
Being afraid that you will never truly connect with others
Seeing yourself as unworthy
Putting yourself in the position of a victim
Seeing no good choices, feeling helpless and powerless
Having people who can dominate and control you
Seeing others as "them," your enemies or adversaries
Being apprehensive about the future

Love solves fear. That's why you can make choices that lead you out of fear into love. If the mind were set up a different way, love wouldn't be the answer. Fear would be like a yellow stain on a linen napkin that you bleach out, leaving a blank. Fear is more than a stain. It's a state of mind that blocks well-being. So well-being, including love, increases as you choose to move out of fear.

Since this is a mind-body book, we've been talking about feedback loops, and just as hunger is part of a feedback loop with satiety, love is on a feedback loop with fear. The same things apply. If the feedback loop is working correctly, you feel love naturally and you act on the impulse you feel. If the feedback loop is distorted—meaning that something has gone wrong with the input or output—the entire situation changes. Consider how simple the mechanism really should be. You want to be loved, so you turn to someone who can love you, and you ask for what you want. Babies and young children have no problem reaching out for a mother's love. They want to be comforted, embraced, reassured, and told that Mommy loves them.

As adults, we find it easy to make this feedback loop a problem. We don't ask for love. Or we do, but we ask the wrong person, who isn't in a position to give us what we want. We divert love into surrogates like making money or acquiring more possessions. In a word, the deep validation that love brings somehow escapes us, and the more we do without it, the more fearful we become that love will never be there. We will wind up unloved and unlovable.

If you can identify with less-than-satisfying love, finding a solution can't help but be important. Even if you feel numb, bored, left out, lonely, or anything else that blocks love, the answer is always self-awareness, because what is holding you back is a mental feedback loop. I realize that people tend to externalize love. There's the fantasy that everything will be perfect once you find "the one." But the solution to finding "the one" is to *be* the one. You must look at the feedback loop inside you and change fear to love. When that happens, the outer situation will change automatically. Even if "the one" doesn't magically appear tomorrow, by returning to a normal, healthy state of love inside yourself, you won't feel so anxious about your fantasy of the perfect soul mate. Any decrease of anxiety is a step toward love.

What Will Make You Happy?

Well-being is the same as happiness, and if polls are to be believed, at least 70 percent of Americans, and often considerably more, report that they are happy. But that's largely a rote response, the thing you are expected to say. When probed in more depth, fewer than a third of Americans are actually thriving, which combines inner and outer satisfactions. The other two-thirds are just getting by or feel that their situation is declining. Although economic downturns play a role, the main reason that people are unhappy is that they haven't found a way to be happy. Human happiness is a goal everyone agrees on, but how to reach it remains a mystery. Let's look at the findings that are most reliable, taken from psychological research in recent years.

The Ingredients of Happiness: What Does the Research Say?

So far as psychologists can tell, making yourself happy depends on some basic, general conditions:

1. You don't settle for unhappiness as a given. Around half of general happiness depends on personal choice, not genes or circumstances.

2. You have material security. Poverty contributes greatly to unhappiness, so it's important to be financially comfortable. Beyond a certain point, however, having more money doesn't increase your happiness. The rich are not uniformly happy, and they are often unhappier than someone with a middle-class income.

3. You try to be happy today, in the here and now. If there's a formula for a happy life, it consists of making each day happy. Fulfillment postponed is fulfillment denied.

4. You stay connected. The happiest people actively spend 1 or 2 hours a day in contact with those they love. They talk on the phone, send e-mails, and text. They don't take their sense of connection for granted.

5. You aren't in physical pain. It's been found that chronic pain is a condition that is difficult, if not impossible, to overcome psychologically. The same is true for depression, which counts as one of the major enemies of happiness because there is no positive way to adapt to it.

6. Each person seems to have a baseline for happiness, a kind of emotional set point. A happy or sad event pushes you away from your set point, but that's rarely permanent. Within six months, almost everyone returns to their set point, feeling about as happy as they did before the sudden upturn or downturn intervened.

This is a fairly meager list, but the field of positive psychology, which studies happiness instead of mental disorders, is still new, and its findings haven't led to a consensus. Yet some key studies seem to agree that most people are bad predictors of what will make them happy. They look to being married, having a child, or getting rich and famous. When the desired thing arrives, however, reality doesn't match expectations. New mothers report that raising a small child is among the greatest stresses in their lives, for example.

Another less-than-positive finding is that permanent happiness may be an illusion. What we should aim for, some psychologists advise, is a state of steady contentment. Moments of happiness come and go. They are unpredictable, and since we are such bad predictors of what will make us happy, it's best not to construct a plan for happiness that won't succeed in the end. We stumble on happiness like stumbling on furniture in the dark, and living with its unpredictability is only realistic.

I find this attitude gloomy and shortsighted. It contradicts the world's wisdom traditions, both Eastern and Western. When Jesus taught that the kingdom of heaven is within, he was pointing out a path to happiness of the highest order. Heaven is a state of joy, and the reason that we stumble upon any experience of happiness, even short of joy, is that we haven't found the right inner path. In the Vedic tradition of India, consciousness itself is imbued with bliss, or *ananda*. We naturally connect to bliss because it exists in our own awareness. If we don't feel blissful, something has blocked the way, and all blockages are in ourselves. Again, an inner path must be found.

To some extent, psychologists are forced to be shortsighted if they themselves haven't found the way to well-being. Understanding the mechanics of human psychology isn't the same as living it. To live in a state of well-being means that you are walking the path of self-awareness. Intellectual understanding helps along the way, of course, but the truth is that what most people need is guidance, not facts. They need to be shown how to evolve and grow, how to overcome inner obstacles, and at the most basic level, how to discover what they really want.

Getting There from Here

As you turn unconscious eating into awareness eating, the next stage—awareness living—isn't far away. Happiness can be woven into every aspect of life once you make new choices. Being able to control how happy or unhappy you are is within your reach, but you need to expand your awareness along the way. Many people try to make themselves happier by choosing more pleasure and less pain. This would seem to be a workable strategy, but it isn't. Let me explain why not at some length.

You have hormones directly connected to the experience of pleasure. In the last chapter I mentioned endorphins, the brain's natural painkillers. Three more hormones can be added to help explain what makes us feel good:

Serotonin
Dopamine
Oxytocin

These are among the most exciting hormones in the public mind because they tell us about basic processes in the brain, holding the key to the world of moods and emotions as viewed by many neuroscientists. Two of the hormones, serotonin and dopamine, also belong to the class of neurotransmitters, which allow two nerve cells to communicate across the gap that separates them, the synapse. These specialized molecules in effect translate thoughts and moods into chemical form, allowing them to communicate—through a complex network of interactions—to the rest of the body. When I say that trillions of cells are eavesdropping on your mind, that largely happens through many kinds of "messenger molecules," as they were originally dubbed.

On the one hand, the link to mental states is strong. This would make us optimistic that by fiddling around with some brain chemicals, happiness is at hand. Serotonin has been tagged as a major player in a person's sense of well-being, while imbalances are associated with depression. (The most popular antidepressants were long thought to help regulate serotonin in the brain, hence their name: selective serotonin reuptake inhibitors [SSRIs]. The basic idea was that in the brains of depressed people, too much serotonin was being reabsorbed, causing a depleted emotional level, and taking an antidepressant corrected the imbalance.)

Dopamine is associated with the good feelings we get when we achieve a success and get what we want. Some people excel at finding rewards from what they achieve, and in these reward-driven individuals, dopamine levels are high. (Addictive drugs like cocaine owe their action to how they affect the dopamine system.) Oxytocin, which was popularly labeled the "love hormone," is associated with sexual orgasms and social bonding—there are high levels in mothers of newborn infants, for example.

On the other hand, happiness isn't chemical. Someone may discover that cocaine gives a burst of incredible happiness, which is chemically induced. But taking cocaine throws off the brain's delicate chemical balance, and after a short while, if addiction sets in, the person discovers that cocaine is a tormenting prison. In a normal life, we can give ourselves bursts of pleasure, but they can't be chemically sustained. Just by looking more closely at the three hormones just introduced, you can see that there is no simple chemical path to happiness.

Consider serotonin and dopamine, which can be found in trace amounts whenever someone feels good about their life. These are complex hormones connected with every other hormone, not to mention more than a dozen other neurotransmitters and more than fifty similar molecules known as peptides. Links extend everywhere, to sleep, appetite, digestion, and stress. It's not just a metaphor to talk about the symphony of hormones. Notice that you can eat something delicious (a pleasurable experience) while feeling guilty at the same time (an unpleasant experience).

There is evidence that if you have a hormonal imbalance involving serotonin and dopamine, your mood can be drastically affected (although the long-held belief that serotonin is the chief actor in depression has been discredited, which says a lot about why antidepressants don't work for many people and in the final analysis may be no better than placebos in their reliability). But much more important is the fact that the mind triggers body chemistry. If you make wrong choices—and choice is a mental process—the bad effects on body chemistry follow.

Here's an example. Imagine yourself driving a car. You're in a hurry, so you have one hand on the wheel and are using the other to eat a sandwich. At the same time you are talking on your cell phone—anyone who has recently taken a taxi in a major city probably saw a cabbie doing all three things at once. In your distraction you almost hit a cyclist on a bike or run a red light. Three things have happened simultaneously:

You were eating unconsciously.
You were giving your mind too many tasks at once.
You wound up in a stressful incident.

At the level of your hormones, all of these things count; they become part of your body chemistry. Although an endocrinologist can separate and isolate each hormone and name its function, in real life there is no such precision. One thing meshes into another. Stress, appetite, digestion, belly fat, mood—there is no strict boundary between them. Brain chemistry tells the tale. You cannot get a happy life by using the formula "more pleasure, less pain," because every state of mind and body is mixed into every other.

A Template for Happiness

Let's step away from the level of chemistry. Chemicals are just footprints telling us where the mind has been. That's why awareness eating works so well—you are controlling the real switch behind the mind-body connection. Happiness is an expanded form of awareness—that same switch has many more functions than eating. "Awareness living" isn't the most elegant of terms, but it tells you what you need to know, as follows:

How Awareness Leads to Happiness

Awareness tells you what is actually going on.
When you know what is going on, you can focus on a solution.
Solutions are a matter of choice.
Making the right choice leads to new chemical messaging.
The new messaging gets imprinted as new pathways in the brain.
The pathways for happiness are as easy to imprint as the pathways for unhappiness.

It's unfortunate that so few people know about the final statement, that making pathways for happiness is as easy as making pathways for unhappiness. They miss this vital point, or never learned it in the first place, because in everyone, old habits, conditioning, memories, prejudices, beliefs, and ego create a fog of illusion. Wandering around in such a fog, people can't be blamed for not recognizing how to solve their problems.

In terms of well-being, we can cut through the fog by looking at what we are hungry for, which starts the process of becoming happy at the first step: Be aware of what's really going on. You can't know what is really going on if you don't pay attention. Your awareness will tell you if you want:

Comfort, security, safety
Love and affection
A sense of belonging
Accomplishment, success, achievement
Self-esteem
Creative expression
Meaning and purpose

I've listed these from the most basic to the most refined needs that exist in human life. Looking at how people respond to their own needs, one sees that under stress—which includes lack of fulfillment—people fall back on their lower needs. Whether or not you actually run back home to reassure yourself that someone loves you, or build a bigger house to feel more important, on the inside everyone will retreat to find the basics of comfort, security, and safety. Where does food belong? At the same lower levels.

Mapping out happiness as a hierarchy of needs—a phrase made famous decades ago by the psychologist Abraham Maslow—makes sense. The insecure Hollywood mogul who insists on living in a huge mansion, the beautiful runway model who secretly binges, the empty-nester who worries constantly about her grown children—in various ways they are all reaching for comfort, security, and safety while being frustrated when they try to fulfill higher needs. But the symphony of hormones should remind us that all our needs are being tended to—or ignored—in a messy chemical soup that reflects how complicated the human mind will always be.

Fortunately, if you attend to higher needs, you won't be compelled to retreat to lower ones. Self-esteem allows you to look at a chocolate cake and say, "I'm not doing that to myself." Creativity fills your day with enough fulfillment that you have no reason to snack out of boredom. Meaning and purpose cancel out the empty feelings that people futilely try to fill by overeating. If you have fulfilled your higher needs, the only reasons that you might gain weight are two: Either you overlooked an aching hunger or you stopped paying attention. Both are lapses of awareness, and bringing your awareness back to what is going on will begin to solve the problem.

Action Step:
An Inventory of Needs

An honest inventory of your needs and how you are fulfilling them will go a long way toward helping you be more aware. Take the seven needs listed on page 192 and rate how well you are doing for each one on a scale from Very Well to Poorly. If you are nervous about taking stock, remember that what you aren't aware of you can't change, and the whole point is change in a positive direction.

Next, list specifically what you are doing to meet the need. Give yourself a suggestion about how to do better. This will give you a connection to what is really going on, and with that awareness, you have begun the process of finding true well-being.

Need #1: *Comfort, security, safety*

I'm doing **Very well About average Below average Poorly**

I tend to this need through the following: _____
_____

(Examples: Owning a house, having a trusted partner/spouse, earning a secure income, living in a safe part of town, taking out insurance, saving for retirement.)

I could do better fulfilling this need by the following:_____
_____

(Use the preceding examples as a guideline—how could you improve each one?)

Need #2: *Love and affection*

I'm doing **Very well About average Below average Poorly**

I tend to this need through the following: _____
_____

(Examples: A loving partner/spouse; close friends; a family where affection is open; being appreciated for your good deeds, service, compassion; believing in God's love.)

I could do better fulfilling this need by the following: _____
_____

(Use the preceding examples as a guideline—how could you improve each one?)

Need #3: A sense of belonging

I'm doing **Very well About average Below average Poorly**

I tend to this need through the following: _____
_____

(Examples: Being part of a community, joining a cause, being of service, bonding with coworkers, working in a cooperative atmosphere, making connections with close friends, mentoring, finding a confidant.)

I could do better fulfilling this need by the following: _____
_____

(Use the preceding examples as a guideline—how could you improve each one?)

Need #4: Accomplishment, success, and achievement

I'm doing **Very well About average Below average Poorly**

I tend to this need through the following: _____
_____

(Examples: Holding a challenging job, being promoted at work, becoming a leader, gaining the respect of others, beating the competition, handling crises, becoming notable in your field, raising your children well.)

I could do better fulfilling this need by the following: _____
_____

(Use the preceding examples as a guideline—how could you improve each one?)

Need #5: *Self-esteem*

I'm doing **Very well About average Below average Poorly**

I tend to this need through the following: _____

_____

   (Examples: Speaking your truth, standing up for yourself, being proud of who you are, appreciating your accomplishments, letting others see who you really are, valuing others as you value yourself, showing dignity.)

I could do better fulfilling this need by the following: _____

_____

   (Use the preceding examples as a guideline—how could you improve each one?)

Need #6: *Creative expression*

I'm doing **Very well About average Below average Poorly**

I tend to this need through the following: _____

_____

   (Examples: Writing, journaling; having creative hobbies like music, painting, and community theater; following your curiosity; making new discoveries; exploring a foreign culture; developing healing and therapeutic skills.)

I could do better fulfilling this need by the following: _____

_____

   (Use the preceding examples as a guideline—how could you improve each one?)

Need #7: *Meaning and purpose*

I'm doing **Very well About average Below average Poorly**

I tend to this need through the following: _____
_____

(Examples: Having a vision and following it, spiritual practice, feeling connected to a higher power, humanitarianism, charity, giving of yourself.)

I could do better fulfilling this need by the following: _____
_____

(Use the preceding examples as a guideline—how could you improve each one?)

Save your inventory and return to it every month. Turn your suggested improvements into real action. At the same time, upgrade your self-rating as you progress, and appreciate how you are contributing to your own well-being.

It's important to realize, as happiness research suggests, that your personal choices matter more than any other factor. Happiness isn't a given, nor is it predetermined. There is no limit to how far our awareness can expand—with that knowledge, the field of positive psychology can make a great contribution. At this moment, however, the project of reaching a state of well-being belongs to you. Don't look upon it as a burden. We all innately follow our own desires, and although pleasure is appealing, we also intuit that life is about much more than a surge of elation now and again. In the next chapter I offer a vision of self-awareness reaching for the highest joy in existence. The same awareness that brings you a happy life has been the guiding light for every wisdom tradition in the world.

Making It Personal:
Emotional Freedom

Having emotions is a natural part of life, something we should celebrate. Having emotional baggage is another story. We've all experienced hurts and wounds in the past. When these hurts and wounds stick with us, we start to owe an emotional debt that is hard to pay—this is our emotional baggage, the dead weight of old experiences. It's crucial to rid yourself of emotional baggage, because worrying about the past blocks your participation in the present. Almost everyone I've ever met who overeats is doing so on behalf of an old self (a discouraged child, an unpopular teenager, a self-conscious young adult) who no longer exists.

To banish these older selves, you must deal with lingering emotional debt. After years of experience with patients, I've found that this can be done without the pain that many people feel when they consider approaching their worst inner pain. It isn't necessary to charge into a minefield; you don't have to brace yourself for a second round of hurt. The process can unfold naturally, and when it does, you will experience relief and a surge of well-being.

The entire exercise goes under the name "Emotional Freedom," and it follows seven steps. Take your time with each step, and don't move on until you feel satisfied that the current step is working for you. (For most people, it helps to have someone else join you in the exercise. Their presence provides reassurance that you aren't alone and unsupported.)

Step #1: Recall an Emotion
With your eyes closed, recall an emotional experience that is causing discomfort. See the circumstances clearly and vividly in your mind. It could be an embarrassing experience or a personal rejection; the feeling could revolve around loss or failure. Don't generalize; be specific. You are recalling an emotional trigger. If your

recollection is too uncomfortable, open your eyes and take a few deep breaths. When you feel less overwhelmed, close your eyes again and proceed.

Step #2: Feel the Emotion in Your Body

Notice where in your body this emotional memory has lodged. For most people, when they bring up a disturbing emotion, a physical sensation of tightness, stiffness, discomfort, or even pain will be felt in the stomach or around the heart. For a smaller number of people the sensation will be felt in the throat or as a headache. Locate where your sensation is occurring.

If at first you don't feel anything, relax, take a breath, and easily tune in to your body. On rare occasions someone may feel numb, which is the sign of a deep emotion that has been tied to fear. But everyone eventually feels something in the body doing this exercise. (I often tell people that an emotion is a thought connected to a sensation.)

Step #3: Label Your Emotion

Now give your emotion a name. Is it fear or anger, sadness or resentment? Most people are surprised to find that they haven't really labeled their emotions in the past. "I feel bad" or "I'm not having a good day" is as far as they get. Being more specific allows you to focus on the emotional baggage you want to release, so take the time to tell yourself exactly what you're feeling.

To help you, here are the most common negative emotions that people carry around:

Anger, hostility, rage

Sadness, grief, sorrow

Envy, jealousy

Anxiety, fear, worry, apprehension

Resentment

Humiliation

Rejection

Shame

Step #4: Express the Experience

Take some paper and a pen. Write down what happened to you during your past experience. Put down in detail how you felt, what other people did, and how you reacted afterward.

When you feel satisfied that you've expressed what the whole thing was about, take a second sheet of paper and retell the same incident from the other person's point of view. Pretend that you are that person. Write down what they were feeling, why they acted as they did, and how they responded afterward. This part is harder than writing down the incident from your point of view, but stick with it—you will be taking a big step toward losing your baggage from the past.

When you are satisfied with what you've written, take a third sheet of paper and relate the same incident as a newspaper reporter would, in the third person. How would an objective observer tell readers about the incident in question? Give the details as objectively and evenhandedly as you can.

This step takes more time than the previous ones, but people enjoy it immensely. They discover that they are no longer trapped in their own point of view. They can suddenly call upon other voices in their head, a new set of eyes, a greater sense of detachment. It's all very freeing.

Step #5: Share the Experience

Now share your experience by reading your three accounts to someone else. In a group setting, which is how I normally lead the exercise, people are eager to share, and the whole tone of the room is lifted, filled with excitement and laughter. The prospect of gaining emotional freedom from their past is exhilarating. So if you are doing the exercise at home, having a partner or a small group really enhances this step.

It works well on your own, however, if you have a good friend or family member you can telephone. Read them your three versions, making sure that they understand why. But don't call the person who caused you the emotional hurt you're recounting. They won't understand and mostly won't cooperate. Ninety percent of the time they won't agree with your version of the event in question; they might deny that it even occurred. So stick with someone who is sympathetic and has your best interests at heart.

Step #6: Create a Ritual

Now it's time to formally let go of your painful experience. Take your written stories and literally let them go. This is done through a ritual where you consign your past to the fire, or symbolically to a higher power that you recognize: the universe, God or the gods, your higher self. You should feel free to devise your own ritual. Set your paper on fire and throw the ashes to the wind or the sea—some people flush them down the toilet. Or they might tear it to pieces and bury them in the backyard.

The ritual is important because it draws a line between your past and who you are right now. If you have fully expressed your old emotion, letting go feels satisfying. But don't hold yourself to a false standard. Letting go takes time and often more than a few repetitions, because some feelings are securely stuck. But they will go; be patient and persistent. Release what you can today. It's normal and natural if you find yourself doing later releases around the same hurt.

Step #7: Celebrate

Once you have released your old story to the universe, celebrate your moment of liberation. You can do this alone or with others, just so long as you appreciate the step you've taken. I find that people often skip this step unless reminded. They don't want to make their emotions a big deal—but in reality they are a big deal. Emotions can trap and bind you, but they can also set you free and change your future.

When you release an old emotion, it's like abandoning a familiar road that has dead-ended. You need to map out a new road or, in this case, a new pathway in the brain. One try doesn't take you all the way down your new road, but it's a start. The famous journey of a thousand miles that begins with one step is yours to travel.

Lightness of Soul

Power Points

- Spiritual experiences depend on the mind-body connection. A spiritual feedback loop sends messages to the brain and every cell in the body.
- The simplest definition of spirituality is self-awareness. Inside yourself is the peace, love, and truth that are attributes of God. When you contact this place, you meet your true self.
- Your true self exists here and now. If you want to meet it, the only requirement is that you be present.
- The present moment never ends, so the choices you make right now affect the rest of your life—life is an unbroken thread of "now" moments.
- To be present, you can learn and practice certain awareness skills.
- When your awareness is fully alive and expanded, you can have the ultimate spiritual experience: "I am the universe." Your being merges with Being itself. Your mind touches the mind of God.

After every other hunger has been satisfied, there is still going to be a spiritual yearning that dwells inside you. It, too, can be satisfied once you know where the right nourishment can be found. The key is inspiration. When you feel inspired, you bring in spirit. When you bring in spirit, you feel inspired. This is the subtlest of feedback loops, yet it connects mind and body in the same way as other feedback loops. When your brain receives spiritual input, it sends messages to every cell in the body. These are chemical messages that decode inner peace and love into a language that can be understood by heart cells, the digestive tract, the skin, and every other organ.

It's not correct to separate spirituality from the body. When you think about God, the soul, or spirit (however you define these terms), you are exposing trillions of cells to a hint of spiritual experience. The experience becomes deeper when thoughts turn into direct contact with the following:

The experience of feeling loved
Communion with nature
Physical sensations of lightness
Being at peace
Expansion of the heart
Feeling unbounded and limitless
A sense of unity with all things
A surge of awe and wonder
The experience of bliss

Everyone has had a glimpse of such experiences—if you recall the last time you were absorbed in the beauty of a sunset or the vastness of the ocean, you were nourishing the feedback loop of spirituality. I believe that everyone is naturally drawn to satisfy their spiritual hunger, which is why we are naturally drawn to these things.

Sometimes it takes only an accident to expose one's inner nature. When I was a boy in India, I fell down while playing, hit my head, and passed out. When I came to, I found myself in a strange reality—the surroundings hadn't changed, but I felt an immense expanse everywhere I looked (unwittingly, I was experiencing something that Don Juan says in one of Carlos Castaneda's books: that for a sorcerer— one who really sees—there is infinity in every direction). The strange expansion of consciousness lasted only a moment or two, and another little boy might have forgotten it immediately. But I was deeply imprinted by it. Looking back, I realize that I had experienced awe for the first time. The rational mind is baffled by awe, and medically speaking, perhaps I was in a swoon or mildly concussed. But rational or not, awe enriches life from the inside, along with wonder, communion, love, and inspiration.

The trail of hormones and brain chemicals that we've been following grows faint in this area. But we know that spiritual experience isn't invisible. There's something real, not just a ghost in the machine. Studies of the brains of Tibetan Buddhist monks indicate that their years of meditation on the value of compassion left physical footprints; there was increased activity in the frontal lobes, where higher values like love and compassion take place. There was also a change of frequency in the region of the delta waves their brains produced; delta waves are associated with deep sleep. Meditation isn't sleep but a state that is paradoxical, in that it combines deep rest with alertness. The chemical trail of meditation also leads to findings about lowered heart rate, decreased stress hormones, and normalized blood pressure. Brain changes include an increase in alpha waves, which are linked to creativity and "aha" moments.

These physical traces indicate that the feedback loop for spirituality is real. But footprints aren't the same as experiencing the journey. To do that, you must transform your state of awareness. When awareness is completely alive, tuning in to the subtlest experiences of love and joy, you have claimed the domain of spirituality. This is the most inspiring state to live in. Reality shifts in radical ways that everyday reality only hints at. A striking image from India's Vedic tradition gives us a clue about what it means to be transformed. It's the image of a clay jug, the kind village women carried to the well for water (and still do in rural India).

The jug's molded sides define the space inside, which isn't very large, and yet all around it, outside the walls, space is immense. Now shatter the jug. The walls are destroyed, but the space inside the jug remains. Only now, instead of seeming to be separate from all the space around it, there is no separation—the space inside the jug merges with infinite space. In the same way, people assume that they are enclosed in the walls of a separate body and a limited mind. But in reality, the separation is artificial. It's literally true that infinity extends all around us even if we don't choose to see it. Nothing divides us from this infinity. Each of us is merged into the whole, and what we prize in our lives—love, creativity, intelligence, truth—can expand without limitation. Human awareness has this capacity—so the mystic tradition in every culture asserts—and the way is always open.

All of us live inside boundaries and at the same time wish, deep down, that we didn't have to. The greatest of mystical poets, Rumi, could see this almost a thousand years ago:

Have you seen the kind
Who settle for less?
Who creep into corners
Just big enough for one?
They are unopened letters
Whose message is this:
Live! Live! Live!

The verse is a passionate plea to the reader, asking for transformation, the kind of transformation that goes from a life of low expectations to one of unbounded life and freedom. Reading Rumi, one feels a tingling sensation that is a hint of how much you and I want to be as free as he is, as passionate and joyous. At the same time, Rumi knows that the voice that calls to us is faint and fragile:

> *Through the night comes a frail, wavering song.*
> *The moment I can't hear it*
> *I will be gone.*

What he is talking about is our link to the source of mind and body. At the deepest level is a state of pure existence—or being— that is the goal of the spiritual journey. When you are connected to your own being, life itself is fulfilling, and inspiration can be found in every moment. Let me explain this a little more.

Spiritual Awareness

Spirituality is about reconnecting with who you really are. At the source, each of us experiences pure being. It's pure because there isn't any content. Being just is. Yet you won't experience this as an empty state like the cold void of outer space. Instead, you find that being is very full. It has infinite possibilities. At this moment you aren't speaking, but if you decide to, there is no limit to the number of sentences you could speak. These sentences aren't programmed into you. They exist as possibilities, and whether you decide to say "To be or not to be, that is the question" or "Let's watch the Nature Channel," you are drawing on the reservoir of infinite potential that exists in your awareness. From that same reservoir you can tap into more than words. There are infinite discoveries to be made, infinite applications of creativity and intelligence.

Once you discover that you are a spiritual being, you will never see yourself any other way. A new self begins to be revealed. It is perfect, lacking nothing in love, beauty, and wisdom. Such a self may seem incredible from where you stand now—skepticism is only natural before the spiritual journey becomes an important part of your life. On the spiritual journey you discover truths hidden from you in everyday life. To use your awareness for anything less is to fall short of your true self.

Up to now, I've focused on how you can use awareness to improve your life. But awareness isn't simply a tool—it's your essence. Human beings aren't machines that learned to think. We are thoughts that learned to make a machine. In other words, the brain serves the mind, and in a natural (but still wondrous) way, you can create a spiritual brain. Exalted as it sounds to have an epiphany, the same brain that learns a foreign language is needed to unfold subtler levels of reality. These levels aren't unknown lands; they exist here and now, only our brains aren't attuned to perceive them. Your life is only as full as your awareness. When you turn your attention to spirituality, you begin to glimpse the unseen—it's not a miracle, just an extension of looking inside yourself.

One obstacle to going beyond limitations is the word *God*. More people today describe themselves as spiritual but not religious. They have walked away from organized religion for one reason or another. An irritated interviewer once challenged me by arguing that "spiritual but not religious" made no sense.

"It does make sense," I countered, "if you define spirituality without arguing over God, as all religions do."

"So what's your definition of spirituality?" he asked.

"It's simple," I said. "Self-awareness. All the promises of religion come true inside us. Spiritual experiences existed long before anyone organized a religion around them. Inside yourself is still the place you have to go." He had no retort.

In the world's wisdom traditions, spirit is located at a subtle level of awareness. The grosser levels of awareness are devoted to objects and events "out there." You use your five senses to navigate the physical world. But there is a finer kind of awareness that navigates the world "in here." You turned to self-awareness at the beginning of this book when you started asking, "What am I hungry for?" Any time you ask yourself about what's going on "in here," you are using self-awareness. Whatever answer comes back, that's who you are at that moment. The inner world exists to provide answers that can't be gotten "out there." The ultimate questions, such as "Who am I?," "Why am I here?," and "What is the meaning of life?," go to the deepest level. The questions are about your true self, which means that you are exercising self-awareness.

We tend to assume that spirituality belongs to saints and devotees of religion—people who surrender their whole being to God. But self-awareness is universal. A spiritual experience happens whenever you are aware of your true self, which is loving and compassionate. Your true self feels safe in the world. In all directions it sees only peace. The constant experience of the true self is bliss, so whenever you feel a surge of joy, that's your true self—for as long as your joy lasts, you have made direct contact. As we all know, joy fades. This isn't a permanent loss, however. You have become detached from your true self, and making contact again is always possible. Every experience of love, bliss, a sense of belonging, inspiration, intuition, insight, and freedom provides a stepping-stone back to your true self.

Spirituality Is Here and Now

To guide you back to your true self, I'm not asking that you undertake a long journey to an unknown destination. The place you want to reach is as close as the present moment. If your true self doesn't exist here and now, it will never be reachable. All choices occur in the present moment, which means that what you are doing right now is the most important action you can take, not the actions you hope or wish to take, or fear or regret taking. The rest of your life is a journey of nothing but present moments.

The present moment is more mysterious than people realize. First of all, you can't pin it down. To illustrate, there is no doubt that you are going to have a new thought in the next few seconds (it's estimated that our minds have a "moment" of thought or feeling every three seconds). When your next thought comes, it will fill the present moment. You'll think a casual thought like "I'm hungry" or a serious thought like "I'm not in the job I really want."

As an experiment, shut your eyes and tell me what your next thought is going to be. If you try it, you'll find that your mind goes blank. You can't grasp the present moment until it arrives, and if you try to force it, there's a mental blank—the present moment refuses to be caught in a net. The mystery of the "now" isn't just a philosophical riddle. It's practical, because in the "now" only two things can happen:

You are fully present. Your true self is you. You feel free and alive. *Or*
You aren't fully present. Old memories, habits, and conditioning block you. You are trapped in a mental fog.

Being able to experience the first state is highly desirable, because the best life is lived as your true self. The second state, sadly, is where almost everyone lives. They only imagine that they are present. To illustrate, I recently saw a woman named Nina who was in her forties and had been married for fifteen years. She had become overweight, and her husband no longer found her attractive. I was surprised to learn that he had come with her but decided to stay in the waiting room while she saw me alone.

"He doesn't think I should bother with all this stuff," Nina said. By *stuff* she meant her constant battle with her weight.

"Did he tell you that today?" I asked.

Nina shook her head. "He didn't have to. I know what he thinks. We don't talk about it."

"Do you talk at all?" I asked.

She shrugged. "We've been married a long time. We've run out of things to talk about, I guess."

"You're clearly unhappy about that," I pointed out. Nina hung her head. I suggested that her marriage had reached an impasse, a block that was holding everything back. Nina nodded, and she told me more about their home life, which revolved around meals, watching TV, and their kids. Between her husband and herself, almost nothing was happening. It was obvious that they were dragging each other down.

She was stuck in a familiar place, which is known as the past. The present moment didn't really exist. It couldn't exist as long as she and her husband filled it with debris from the past—old arguments not settled, emotions not expressed, opinions quashed, and so on. They had "solved" their problems by turning the present moment into a dead zone. It felt empty, but at least they weren't feeling much pain.

"You can get out of this trap," I said. "No one set it but yourself."

Nina protested. "You don't have to live with him."

"You're right. I've never even met your husband. I'm sure you have a lot of grievances you could air. If you told him everything that's wrong with him, your marriage, and all the rest of it, we could spend hours here. But the answer really does lie with you," I said. "You are absent right now from your own life, when what you desperately need is to be present."

I asked Nina to close her eyes and sit quietly. Then I led her through a simple exercise.

"Ask yourself if you are being aware right now. Are you?" Nina nodded. "Okay," I said. "What are you aware of? Don't put it into words. Just check yourself. Check your body. Do you feel any sensations? Check your mood. Look quietly at your mind. When you've finished checking in, open your eyes."

After a moment she was looking at me again. I asked her to describe her inner inventory. Nina said that her mood was down, and yet her body felt pretty good. There was something even nicer. It was a lovely spring day, and I had the window open. A sea breeze was coming in, and with it the faint smell of the ocean.

"I was so caught up in my problems," Nina said, "that I didn't notice how nice a day it is. But once I felt the breeze over my skin, I began to relax, and then I noticed."

"Perfect," I said with enthusiasm. "To be in the present moment, you need to be present. Everything that life has to offer comes to us through our awareness. When you are present, you drink in everything that your mind, body, and environment are telling you. Without awareness, your life tells you nothing, because you are only aware of the habits and rituals that get you through the day."

There was more to say, but the key thing is that Nina left promising to repeat the simple awareness exercise she had just learned. Her marriage could improve—along with a host of other issues—only if she started to be present. Nothing would change, however, if she kept being an internal defector.

Your true self wants to connect with you. If you couldn't contact your true self, there would be no magic in the present moment. It would be just another tick-tock on the clock, another silent numeral on your digital watch. What tells us that the present moment contains magic is that you can only love, feel joy, and be inspired here and now. The intensity of life happens only in the present.

Don't regret the fact that you haven't been living in the present. The universe is set up to exemplify a truth stated by the great quantum physicist Erwin Schrödinger: "The present is the only thing that has no end." This is more than an interesting point in physics; it's the doorway to a kind of practical immortality, the timeless domain where every possibility exists here and now.

Skills in Awareness

The present moment requires you to be aware of it, but is that enough? People who have lost their memory to Alzheimer's disease or amnesia can't connect with their past. They live in the present, it could be said, and yet they suffer. It's true that blank awareness has nothing to offer. You have to participate in your own consciousness. Most people spend hardly a minute dwelling in the deep silence and peace that exists inside them; it is totally foreign territory. But the world's wisdom traditions discovered that awareness possesses hidden advantages. These advantages are tucked away in silence, and yet we all have them.

If you delve into our own awareness, you will notice the following:

- Ever since you were a child, your mind has favored moving forward over inertia. It doesn't like being stuck.
- Once it begins, evolution accelerates its pace.
- Consciousness naturally expands. The path of desire is fueled by wanting more.
- The better you know yourself, the better your life becomes.
- Positive intentions are supported more than negative intentions.
- Individual consciousness is connected to a higher consciousness, which we sense as a feeling of belonging to a higher purpose.

You alone are the explorer of your inner world. To test whether these advantages actually exist is the path of self-awareness. The feedback loop may be weak when you start. You haven't thought about how to grow and evolve—too much time was gobbled up by earning a living, raising a family, and exploring the world "out there." Even so, you have been building a self all your life, and the process took place in awareness.

Now you can become skilled at building the self you actually want. It will expand everything on the list:

You will favor moving forward every day.

Your personal growth will accelerate.

The better you know yourself, the more you will cherish your life.

You will become more positive as self-judgment falls away, and this positivity will be reflected in your outer life.

You will feel connected to a higher vision of life and a higher power that makes your vision come true.

These are practical things, markers on the spiritual journey that you reach in real life. I measure my progress by them every day. I am moving forward if I feel more compassion, less blame, and greater calmness. My personal growth is accelerating when a goal that I thought would take years—such as dropping the need for anger—arrives much sooner. I firmly believe in being as down-to-earth as possible. There have been moments when I was sitting on the fast train from New York to Boston and gazing out at the gray landscape whizzing by; I merged into it, feeling as if Deepak had vanished and there was only Being, the peace of pure existence. These privileged moments are the kind of markers I'm talking about.

Spirituality has languished too long as a set of beautiful ideals. Only the type of spirituality that creates real change is useful. By its nature, awareness is life-supporting—miraculous as the mind is, arising from an organ that weighs 3 pounds and is the consistency of cold oatmeal, it is responsible for basic needs like sustaining the body and ensuring your survival. The greatest gift you can give yourself is to be present, because then the perfect match between awareness and the "now" is made.

I've painted a glowing picture, but in practice, what should you do?

Once you see the value of being present, you can acquire the skills necessary to get there. These skills train your brain to be present, and as you reinforce new pathways, being present gets easier and easier, until one day it feels completely natural—indeed, to be present is much easier than surrounding yourself with the fog of illusion. Dwelling on the past or anticipating the future is totally illusory. The past and the future don't exist. Only the "now" exists, and therefore it's the home you were born to live in.

Action Step:
How to Acquire Awareness Skills

Your brain was designed to respond to spiritual experiences. When you feel inspired or filled with wonder, that experience is processed in the brain. But you can also train your brain to be much more receptive to spiritual input. We'll cover four of the most important skills in awareness:

Being centered
Paying attention
Holding focus
Diving deeper

Skill #1: *Being Centered*

Being centered is the most basic awareness skill. Most people can't be in the present because they are too busy being somewhere else.

They are distracted by the world "out there," which is filled with constant activity. But haven't you noticed certain people who have the following qualities?:

They know who they are.
They focus sharply on the task at hand.
They seem self-possessed and comfortable with who they are.
They listen closely.
They don't crave the approval of others or fear disapproval.
They grow calm in a crisis rather than flustered or panicky.

Such a person is centered. They are comfortable being here instead of being somewhere else. In a society that lavishes everyone with distractions of every kind, being centered takes effort. You must train yourself not to be distracted. If you don't, there will always be something new—a phone call, a movie, a crisis at home, a deadline at work—to pull you out of yourself. But if you remain in yourself, you will handle your life better, including those aspects "out there" that need answers and solutions.

Does all of this run the danger of being self-centered? There are critics who think so, although I think the specter of the "me" generation isn't hovering over us here. Being self-centered is the same as rampant egotism, where what counts first and foremost is myself and what I want. Ultimately, such a state is a form of insecurity, while being centered is the opposite. People who are secure in themselves tend to be emotionally flexible and caring of others. Egotists have brittle boundaries; they can't reach out to others (and therefore pretend that reaching out isn't worthwhile).

Being centered saves a lot of trouble. Here's a recent real-life example. A friend of mine went to get cash from an ATM, only to discover that she was overdrawn on her account. She was baffled and a bit shocked, but she was late for an appointment, so she rushed home, found the checkbook from another account, and hurried back to the bank, which was now closed. She stuffed the check into an ATM envelope and dashed off to make her appointment.

The next day she went to the ATM for cash, only to discover that she was still overdrawn. Fuming at the bank's mistake, she confronted the manager, who showed her the check she had deposited. She had forgotten to sign it. Embarrassed, she added her signature, and the incident was over. It seems normal enough to be shocked by an overdraft you didn't expect, but if my friend hadn't been so frazzled, she would have signed the check and avoided all the stress and wasted time. She lost her center. A small incident, but multiply it by all the times that you find yourself thrown off your center—for most people, everyday stress will do it. They don't even notice what has happened, because they are so used to having their awareness be jerked here and there by external events.

Being centered comes naturally once you put your mind to it. First, stop doing the things that defeat being centered:

- Don't multitask. Focus on the moment at hand.
- Resist being distracted. If someone needs to interact with you at work, for instance, close the door, turn off the phone, and have your computer screen go black. Let the person see that you are focused on them. People can tell if you aren't interested in them, and one of the surest signs is silent impatience while you wait to say what you have to say. Avoid the other obvious signs of a lack of interest, such as tapping your pencil, fidgeting, interrupting others before they finish, or glancing out the window.
- Don't scatter your attention randomly. Manage your mental time efficiently, so that you can be alone for serious thinking. Devote time to others without feeling that you are being pulled away from what you're really interested in.

Avoiding these missteps and bad habits will go a long way in your relationship with others. But you also need the positive experience of being centered. It begins when you are alone. In a quiet place, close your eyes, take a deep breath, and go inward. Place your attention on your heart, in the center of your chest. Sit quietly, and easily let your attention remain there. If it is pulled away by random thoughts, re-center as soon as you notice what has happened. After a few minutes, open your eyes. For the next half hour or so, observe yourself to see if you remain centered. Don't instantly throw yourself into external demands.

If you repeat this practice several times a day, you will start to learn the difference between being centered and not. With repetition you train your brain, and in turn your involuntary nervous system, to prefer a calm, quiet, centered state. This preference brings along lower blood pressure, decreased stress response, and slower heart rate. You aren't inert and unresponsive; nor are you forcing your attention to stay in the middle of your chest. The state you want is more responsive, in fact, because your awareness is closer to home, allowing you to access answers without outer distractions.

Skill #2: *Paying Attention*

Attention is important, because whatever you pay attention to grows. If you focus on your job, your relationship, or a favorite hobby, your attention nourishes that feedback loop. (When an unhappy wife complains that her husband doesn't pay attention to her, he misses the point if he replies, "But I got you this house and everything you wanted." Attention is the most personal and precious thing you can give.) Attention can't be faked or forced. When a schoolteacher scolds an unruly class with, "Pay attention, people!" he may get results for a minute or two, but the demand loses its effect quickly. Asking a restless mind to settle down and pay attention is even more futile. The secret is to know how attention really works.

Attention is focused awareness. The first requirement is being centered, as we've just covered, because you have to be here in the first place. Second, your awareness focuses naturally when you have a desire. We focus on what we want. Third, attention works best when combined with intention—finding a way to fulfill your desire. When the three ingredients come together—you are centered, you have a desire, you have an intent to fulfill your desire—attention becomes extremely powerful. The tale is told by anyone who has fallen in love at first sight; it's the definition of laser focus. But for some people the same focused attention applies to ambition, money, and power.

Attention becomes spiritual when you focus on objects of inner desire. Almost everyone has wondered, "Who am I?," but the ones who actually find out are driven by a desire to know. This desire is as strong as other people's desire for more money, status, and power. If you ask spiritual questions casually, they amount to little. God could send you a text message with the answers and it wouldn't change your life. The whole spiritual path must be driven by desire. Let's say that you experience a moment of inner peace that has arrived without expectation. It's just there, appearing in the midst of an ordinary day.

You might casually notice it, or a train of thought could begin, as follows:

I'm at peace. How unusual. I like this.

I wonder where it came from.

I want to find out, because it would be good to be at peace more often.

I'm going to follow this experience up. It's too valuable to forget.

This is a natural train of thought, and every spiritual person I know has followed it, not necessarily from a moment of inner peace. Some experience sudden joy; others felt protected and looked after; a few sensed a divine presence that caught them totally by surprise. What they had in common was that they really paid attention to their experience. The process can be simplified into three steps. The next time you have an inner experience of peace, joy, love, inspiration, or insight, pause for a moment:

Step 1: Notice what is happening. Sit quietly without distraction. Soak up the experience without commenting or interrupting it.

Step 2: As the moment fades, don't rush away from it. Consider how significant it is. Put the significance into context, reflecting on how different you feel from your ordinary self.

Step 3: Make the experience valuable. Consider how transformed your life would be if you could repeat the experience. Even more, think about a life filled with joy, peace, and love. See it in your mind's eye; feel how beautiful your life would become.

In these three steps you are activating the emotional brain and the cortex, or higher brain—the first by fully feeling your experience, the second by applying thought and reflection. This is how dreams come true. You combine a vision of possibilities with the kind of focused intention that creates new pathways in the brain. The world "in here" is always connected to the world "out there." You can't seize an opportunity without being aware of it; you can't nourish a new possibility without wanting to. When awareness, desire, and intention come together, you are mastering the skill of attention.

Skill #3: *Holding Focus*

When you desire something, keeping focused on it comes naturally. But it's harder to talk about focus in spiritual terms. God, the soul, spirit, or a higher power are vague images in most people's minds.

Many cling to a Sunday school picture of God as a white-bearded patriarch sitting above the clouds, in large part because it's a visual image that can be vividly seen. But to focus on God as a person doesn't get at reality, nor does imagining your soul as a wispy ghost in the vicinity of your heart. Spiritual values are invisible and intangible, yet they come to life in your awareness.

To make spiritual values real, you must use a different kind of focus, known as *clear intention*. Knowing what you want, uncomplicated by confusion, is a clear intention. Your body obeys clear intentions more easily than confused intentions. Just look at the body language of someone who can't wait to get to the golf course as opposed to someone being dragged to church. Every time you hesitate or feel mixed emotions, your intention is no longer clear. It's the difference between running a marathon burning to win and running the same marathon worrying that you might collapse halfway through. The brain is thrown off by mixed messages, even when they are subtle. For example, if you know how to make an omelet, it will generally take less than two minutes from start to finish. But try timing yourself against the clock, setting a deadline of two minutes. You'll find yourself fumbling over easy steps, and at the very least your mind will be divided between making the omelet and keeping your eye on the clock.

The problem of mixed motives applies to spiritual matters and leads to much frustration. Consider the act of prayer. People pray under many different circumstances: some of them quite desperate, when the mind is agitated, and some of them quite peaceful, when the mind calmly turns to God. There are prayers for redemption, forgiveness, or healing—or, if you happen to be ten years old, for a new bike. People make bargains in their prayers: "God, if you give me what I want, I promise to be good" is a well-tried formula. The fact that some prayers are answered while many are ignored leads to enormous confusion and frustration. But in terms of awareness, prayer can't be expected to work if your intention isn't clear. In every area of life, intentions become murky when you:

Don't really know what you want
Think you don't deserve to get what you want
Feel skeptical that any result will come
Have mixed motives
Experience inner conflict

Prayer is a big subject, and I'm not passing judgment on whether it works (given a clear connection to your true self, I believe that prayers—or any clear intention—can come true). But the lines of communication are cut off when you send a confused message. With clarity comes focus, and when you are focused, the power of awareness is activated.

The secret to holding focus is to make it effortless. The image of a genius with furrowed brow concentrating like mad is the wrong image. Awareness likes to be focused when it is pleased—that's why two people in love can't tear their eyes off each other. They drink each other in; there's no effort involved. So apply your focus to the things that charm you in spiritual life. For me, the poetry of Rumi has been fascinating for thirty years because I love the feeling it gives me. Inspiring spiritual writings all have the same effect on me, as they do for most people once they remember to start reading. In a more expanded definition, you can find spiritual pleasure anywhere—a tropical sunset, the sight of children at play, the serenity in the face of someone as they sleep.

Focus is effortless but not passive. When you truly focus on a spiritual experience, the following happens:

You relax into a receptive state.
You are quiet inside.

The experience is allowed to sink in.

You are filled with a subtle feeling of beauty, pleasure, wonder, or love.

You appreciate this feeling and allow it to linger.

In short, this is one of the gentlest skills in awareness, and one of the most pleasing.

Skill #4: *Diving Deeper*

When I think of my mind, I see the image of a river. On the surface there are lapping waves, and the current flows quickly. Dive beneath the surface and the same river flows more slowly; there are no waves agitating the water. Keep diving, and the water slows even more, until at the bottom there is hardly any motion at all. Yet it's all the same river. Most people spend 90 percent of their waking hours at the surface of the mind, which is tossed and turned by daily events. It would be easy to believe that this restless activity *is* the mind. There is nothing else until you dive deeper and experience it.

We've all had moments when our minds grew more peaceful—millions of people go on vacation just to find this experience. But the world's wisdom traditions don't consider peace and calm a vacation. They teach that the nature of the mind is silent, vast, and calm. The mind's activity—meaning all the thoughts and feelings you could possibly have—is secondary. The silent mind is primary. But why? You won't know the value of silence until you acquire the skill to get there and explore it on your own. Children in kindergarten are told to put their heads down for a few minutes every afternoon. You probably remember how impatient this made you, how quickly you wanted to get back to playing and running around.

In adults, this same impatience has worn a deep groove. We resist being still because what we know is activity, a constant state of mental churning. If the nature of the mind is silent, calm, and peaceful, it's not part of our experience. Millions of people in the West have heard of meditation by now. A large number have given it a try. Life is stressful and hectic enough that getting a short respite every day sounds appealing. But the spiritual teacher J. Krishnamurti said something important when he declared that true meditation lasts twenty-four hours a day. True meditation occurs when you dive deep into your mind and stay there.

Diving deeper brings you closer to your source. At the mind's source is creativity, intelligence, peace, and bliss. You don't have to work to achieve these things. They are part of the landscape. As the saying goes, they come with the territory. Meditation allows you to find the territory in the first place. A glimpse isn't hard to find, and with repetition, the glimpse grows into a view. Your mind will like what it sees, and so the desire to dive deeper increases on its own.

To dive deeper right this minute, here's a simple breath meditation. Sit quietly by yourself. Make sure that you won't be disturbed. Close your eyes for a moment to clear your mind and make it receptive. Now place your attention on the tip of your nose. Feel the air gently going in and out as you breathe. Do this for 10 minutes. If your attention strays from the tip of your nose—as it naturally will—easily bring it back. Don't force your attention; don't try to control your breathing. Just be natural and easy.

Before you open your eyes, sit and appreciate where you are inside. Let the feeling sink in—just be with it. Now open your eyes and go about your day. Almost everyone will find that the effects of this simple meditation linger for a while. Colors seem a bit more vivid, or sounds seem clearer. There's a sense of calm inside and less tendency to be pulled out into activity. If your day is frantic and you plunge quickly back into it, this lingering will be slight. But meditate twice a day for 10 to 20 minutes, and then you will begin to taste a lasting difference.

Silence would have little use except as a kind of inner vacation if it didn't change outer life. That's the ultimate measure. By keeping up a faithful meditation schedule for a month, you are in a position to ask yourself the following questions:

A Meditation Inventory

Do I feel lighter?

Do I have more energy?

Am I more settled?

Are the hard things getting easier?

Has my mood improved?

Is my stress level lower?

Have I had some inspiring moments?

Do I feel more grateful?

Do I appreciate my life more?

Am I getting closer to those I love?

Do I feel that I belong?

Am I judging myself—and others—less than I used to?

Am I more comfortable inside myself?

Do I have inner peace?

This inventory is detailed. It has to be, because whenever someone says, "I tried meditating for a while, but it dropped away," they usually have no specific reason for quitting. A new habit didn't take hold; old habits did. But if you go through the inventory item by item, you'll realize that meditation isn't about simply feeling a bit calmer. It's about activating the whole mind, and the whole mind touches every aspect of your life.

Using these four skills, you can make the spiritual path practical.

Transformation comes within reach. It's no longer a dream or a far-away vision inspired by scriptures and poetry. The greatest miracles are achieved by accepting the gift of awareness that you were born with. It may seem as if we've wandered a long way from where we began. Overeating was the original problem, which most of us would consider important to solve but mundane. Yet the solution—awareness eating—had a long reach. It expanded into awareness living, and the most inspiring way to live is spiritually. The themes of lightness, purity, energy, and balance apply to lightness of soul and purity of heart, the balance of inner and outer, and the energy to pursue your highest fulfillment.

It spoils life to sit in the corner like one of Rumi's unopened letters. For me, it takes only a reminder from Rumi to return to the meaning of life:

This day knows itself
Beyond what words can tell,
Like passing a cup on which is written,
Life is mine, but not mine.

Life belongs to each of us, but we also belong to life. Every moment when you feel fulfilled, you are bringing a cosmic impulse to fruition. In the present moment a cup is passed back and forth. You hold it in your hands for the briefest second before handing it back to the universe. The greatest miracle is that when you receive it again, the cup is always full, ready to be savored anew.

Making It Personal:
How to Be Whole—A Seven-Day Meditation

At the beginning of this book I spoke about joining a ground-swell of change. It made a big difference in my lifestyle when I joined it; I became more aware of my eating, and that small step led to a deeper understanding of what "nourishment" really means for mind, body, and soul.

But there is another groundswell of change that reaches even further, beyond the boundary of one person's life—the movement for finding a holistic way to live. This movement is global and affects everyone, because with the ecology in peril and the pressure of overpopulation, trying to live as we have in the past isn't possible. Life sustains itself, and yet human beings are the caretakers of life. We are called upon to sustain the environment, and yet the way forward isn't clear by any means.

Living holistically means that you feel connected to everything else. A tree in the Amazon exhales oxygen, which you need in order to live, while you exhale carbon dioxide, which that tree needs in order to live. The virus that makes a child sick in China travels by jet to reach the doorstep of another child somewhere else in the world. Water, food, and air are no longer local needs. They nourish the body of the planet. For the individual, a holistic lifestyle must still bring happiness. We aren't asked to be monks and nuns renouncing our well-being so that Mother Earth can get better. The two are complementary. You can be happy and at the same time promote the well-being of all life.

Most of the themes you've practiced in this book apply to holistic living, especially purity and balance. Gobbling up the planet's limited resources is unbalanced. Fouling the atmosphere with pollutants is impure. Why do we continue to do what we know is obviously wrong? Because we are attached to being happy, and the old template for happiness depends on being a consumer who craves more of everything, disposes waste products carelessly, focuses on "I, me, and mine" without regard for the whole human family, and lives for the moment, leaving the future to take care of itself.

I believe that your life can be just as happy by aiming higher. Fulfillment will always be the key. But inner fulfillment is much more satisfying than the promise of happiness based on endless consumption. I'd like to offer a new template for happiness to replace the old one. You are asked to find fulfillment every day starting from "in here." You won't be joining a cause or crusade. Instead, you will be making a connection. This connection starts with yourself and then spreads outward.

Below is a seven-day meditation that is effortless but full of meaning. It's been successful and popular with hundreds of people who began following it at the Chopra Center. Read the vision for each day, and then spend the time to practice that day's meditation. A separate mantra assigned to each day is derived from the Vedic tradition of India—using it is optional but recommended, since mantras settle the mind into a deeper place.

You are already connected to all life on earth—that's a given—and now it's time to actually feel the connection and let it sink into your awareness. Many people have called for a shift in consciousness and a new paradigm for the future. Here's a way to answer that call personally.

Sunday, Day 1
Perfect Health

There exists in everyone's awareness a place that is free from disease, that never feels pain, that is joyful and vibrant. When you journey to this place, the limitations we commonly accept cease to exist. If the mind-body connection is strong, awareness can be converted into perfect health. This isn't a dream. In the body's feedback loop, every intangible thought, feeling, and sensation is converted into chemical or electrical signals. Awareness is constantly affecting the body. Therefore, it's only reasonable to believe that negative messaging has negative consequences for health, while positive messaging has the opposite effect.

Perfect health is the norm of every cell. Imperfections are healed or the cell dies. If it is forced to exist in an imperfect state, a cell can adapt with extraordinary flexibility—that's how the heart manages to function for years even with decreased oxygen from blocked coronary arteries, for example. But if the imbalanced state lasts long enough, cells, tissues, and organs die. Since perfect health is the norm for your cells, it should be the norm for you as the person who sends every message to those cells. How you intervene depends on the choices you make. Every intervention for good supports the body's perfect health; every negative intervention puts stress on the body and pushes it, either a little bit or a lot, toward ill health.

It has taken decades for modern medicine to recognize the mind-body connection, and since doctors are still trained only to treat isolated parts of the body, being healthy is your responsibility. Raising this to perfect health demands more awareness. This book has described what "awareness living" can do for you. Having all the tools is important. But you must pick up and use the tools. It's easy to settle for less, and when your expectations drop, old patterns pop up out of nowhere, offering the course of least resistance.

What fuels a conscious way of life is inspiration, and inspiration comes from within. It doesn't arrive in the form of uplifting messages—although these are good in their own right—but from a settled state of being centered and at home within yourself. Protected from the agitations of stress and outer pressure, you will find it easier to follow your new vision of life. A calm voice will show you how to do what you know is right for you. This becomes the course of least resistance, not dropping back into bad habits. In today's meditation, and all the ones that follow, the goal is simple: the next thing you want to do will be the best thing you can do for yourself.

As you begin your first day's meditation, contemplate this centering thought: *I commit to living in perfect health.*

To begin, find a comfortable position, placing your hands gently in your lap and closing your eyes. Observe the inflow and outflow of your breath. With each inhalation and exhalation, allow yourself to become more relaxed, more comfortable, more at ease.

The mantra: Now, gently introduce the mantra that allows you to connect to this memory of wholeness, repeating it mentally and allowing it to flow with effortless ease: *Om Bhavam Namah,* which means "I am absolute existence. I am a field of all possibilities."

Silently repeat it with your eyes closed. Whenever you find yourself distracted by thoughts, sensations in your body, or noises in the environment, simply return your attention to mentally repeating the mantra.

Continue with your meditation. When you think that about 10 minutes have passed, take a peek at your watch or clock. If you have more time left, close your eyes and continue with the mantra. If the 10 minutes are up, then it's time to release the mantra. Gently bring your awareness back into your body. Take a moment to rest, inhaling and exhaling slowly and deeply. When you feel ready, gently open your eyes.

Follow through: As you continue with your day, carry with you the knowledge that simply with a change of mind, you can change your life. Return occasionally to this centering thought: *I am creating perfect health with every choice. I am creating perfect health with every choice.*

Monday, Day 2
The Wisdom of Your Body

Each of us possesses an inner wisdom that isn't reflected in our daily thoughts, which are mostly occupied with the business of living. This wisdom is rooted in the body. While human beings fight and disagree, trillions of cells synchronize every biological process down to the thousandth of a second. While the ego drives us to fulfill self-centered ambitions, every part of the body instinctively works in concert, always looking out for the whole. Cells don't know how to be selfish, and if they happen to forget the well-being of the entire body, such cells become malignant. Pursuing their own expansion at any cost, they invade other parts of the body, only to discover in the end that their only reward is death.

You've been learning how to obey the wisdom of your body over many pages. When you trust your body completely, you stop interfering with its wisdom. You stop overloading it with stress, lack of sleep, a bad diet, and hours a day of total inactivity with intermittent bursts of overactivity. We're all embedded in a materialistic worldview, and for a long time a notion like the wisdom of the body was dismissed—as it still is in some quarters—as unscientific. But there is no need to replow that field. The mind-body connection is a scientific certainty, and the major breakthrough came from researchers who showed that the chemical messages sent back and forth by brain cells were found in the digestive tract, immune system, and skin. The brain was no longer the sole seat of intelligence. Instead, intelligence was like a river coursing through every tissue. It was entirely accurate to refer to the immune system as a floating brain and to consider gut feelings as legitimate as emotions "in your head."

The biochemistry of intuition and insight hasn't emerged yet, or the inner river that makes humans so curious and creative. But it is certain that the mind-body connection will be involved—all that is needed is to find subtler ways of observing it. In the world's wisdom traditions, the body's wisdom doesn't need to be justified, as if it were ever in doubt. Wisdom exists in a state of unity already. The body is seen as one component in the cosmic dance, and its display of intelligence derives from a field of intelligence that organizes all of creation. This is a spiritual view, although if you could ask a cell where it came from, it would point to the whole body as a matter of course—a heart or liver cell doesn't believe for an instant that its life is isolated, separate, or accidental. Being a single cell in the body of the universe, which each of us is, has the same basis. If you could be as wise as your body, everything in your life would be in harmony with everything else. Meditation is a powerful way to bridge the gap between our imperfect self-image and the perfection that comes effortlessly to our bodies.

As you begin meditation, contemplate this centering thought: *I trust the wisdom of my body.*

Begin your meditation, following the instructions from Day 1.

The mantra: Now, gently introduce the mantra. It is the sound, *Shyam,* that is associated with intuition and inner wisdom. It is pronounced "shi-um."

Follow through: As you continue with your day, listen for your intuition and contemplate this centering thought: *My mind and body are in perfect sync. My mind and body are in perfect sync.*

Tuesday, Day 3
Restoring Balance

The key to restoring balance and keeping our ideal weight is to expand our awareness from unconscious habits to self-aware choices. Whenever we have an experience, the mind is in one of three states: unconscious, aware, or self-aware. The mind's two main modes of operation, unconscious and aware, are highly developed. When acting in the unconscious mode, the brain is able to take care of the body without needing specific detailed instructions, processing the five senses to keep us aware of our inner and outer worlds. However, in the unconscious state, health and well-being are generally left to chance, and the critical mind-body feedback loop operates automatically without any awareness.

Consider this example: If you get to the break room at work and pour your third cup of coffee of the day without thinking, you're doing something unconsciously, which is the mode of operation that underlies habits. If you see yourself reaching for the coffee urn, then you are aware. Now you see the last muffin left out for the taking. Self-awareness can also step in. In that moment, you can ask, "What am I getting out of this?" When we begin to ask ourselves questions, reflecting on our behaviors, looking at the larger picture, and then inviting the answers to come to us, we move into the place of self-awareness. Being self-aware, you begin to pay attention to the one who is aware, the true self. The true self is where values, meaning, purpose, and answers come from.

Self-awareness moves us beyond the old, well-worn pathways in the brain that support fixed, unconscious habits. Imagine a situation in which you are angry. In this instance, when you recognize, "I'm angry," you are having an aware thought. But knowing where your anger comes from invites a component of self-awareness into the situation, allowing you to recognize a pattern of behavior. You realize that old habits—past outbursts, for example—likely haven't served you well, and you begin to take steps to transcend those habitual responses.

Reality shifts when self-awareness enters, and we start to take control with the help of our spirit. Becoming self-aware opens the door to lasting change and empowers us to make the most nourishing choices in every moment.

Here's the centering thought for today's meditation: *With awareness, I create healthy habits.*

Begin your meditation, following the instructions from Day 1.

The mantra: Now, gently introduce today's mantra. It is *Om Kriyam Namah.* (*Kriyam* is pronounced "kree-yum.") This translates as "My actions are aligned with cosmic law."

Follow through: As you continue with your day, contemplate this centering thought: *With awareness, I create healthy habits. With awareness, I create healthy habits.*

Wednesday, Day 4
Breathing for Balance

All living beings are enlivened by breathing, the exchange of life-supporting atoms in the atmosphere or ocean. In the Indian tradition, breathing has a subtler level connected with the life force, or *prana*. In this ancient model, prana pulses through the body and gives us life. In Sanskrit, *prana* simply means "breath," and on that basis—without needing to accept the underlying notion of a life force—many exercises have been devised that use breathing to make a person feel calm, centered, and balanced. These subjective feelings have also been connected to physical benefits such as lower blood pressure and heart rate.

People also report that prana exercises give them increased energy during the day. In the West, studies of the "subtle body" are rare, because there isn't a match between ancient and modern models. Even so, yoga is based on an ancient model, and thousands of people benefit from it without having to adopt a different worldview. Prana is thought to activate all the life forces in the body. And, while prana energizes us in the form of breath, any form of energy—light, heat, electricity—is associated with prana, just as in modern medicine the brain's activity depends on a merging of chemical and electrical processes, with nourishment derived from food and oxygen.

In the yogic tradition there are elaborate practices for controlling the flow of prana, but in Western terms, the whole point is to provide better input into the mind-body connection. Mental clarity and energy are essential to listening to your body. So prana functions in the Indian system as a kind of biofeedback. As you've discovered in this book, awareness serves the same purpose. There is a link with meditation here. The more you practice being connected with your breath, the more spontaneously you move into a settled state of awareness—conscious breathing brings the mind back to itself.

Here's the centering thought for today's meditation: *I am one with the breath of life.*

Begin the meditation, following the instructions from Day 1.

The mantra: Now, gently introduce today's mantra. It is *So Hum*, which means, "I am."

Follow through: As you continue with your day, contemplate this centering thought: *I am sustained by the breath of life. I am sustained by the breath of life.*

Thursday, Day 5
Eating for Balance

Eating is a daily activity, but there is a deeper significance to food. In the West we've studied food in terms of measurable nutrition— calories, proteins, fats, vitamins, and so on—while from a holistic viewpoint you are what you eat. Food is just about the energy our bodies extract from it. The body converts food into thoughts, feelings, sensations, moods, and everything else in the complexity of the mind-body system. Therefore, food is merged with consciousness, intelligence, and every choice you make in a day. When you eat natural, whole foods and drink clean, fresh water, you enhance the life-giving energy that knits thousands of processes into a whole person.

In the medical system of Ayurveda from India, nourishment is approached holistically to reach a state of dynamic balance. Centuries later, Western research confirms the chemical bond that unites food and the brain, giving physical proof that in terms of the messages circulating throughout the body, "you are what you eat" was right all along. The most basic message that food sends comes from the act of eating. If you eat in a rush, paying no attention to your food, offering no gratitude but merely stoking your engine, there is no effect on the calories and nutrients that the food contains. There's a big change, however, in your experience. When you take the first bite, your body receives a rush of information, primarily through taste but also through your thoughts, feelings, mood, and expectations. "I really shouldn't be eating this" sends a different message from "I'm really doing myself some good."

You can make eating an optimal experience, and when you do, not just your food but the whole experience gets metabolized.

It's important to appreciate and celebrate food for its holistic value. Eating with awareness, sitting in a warm atmosphere with loved ones, and making the meal a zone for positive exchanges will set the stage for the best experience. The meal will be in harmony with your body. You will be eating for fulfillment.

Here's the centering thought for today's meditation: *I choose foods that help me thrive.*

Begin your meditation, following the instructions from Day 1.

The mantra: Now, gently introduce the mantra, *Om Vardhanam Namah*, which means, "I nourish the universe and the universe nourishes me."

Follow through: As you continue with your day, contemplate this centering thought: *I eat to nourish mind, body, and spirit. I eat to nourish mind, body, and spirit.*

Friday, Day 6
Moving for Balance

Your body wants to move, and if you move in accord with your own nature, you will receive almost all the benefits of organized exercise. Movement is personal. The most advanced research in sports science reveals that not everyone benefits the same from doing exercise—improvements in blood oxygen and added strength vary enormously. For the most part, your body will tell you how to be active. There's a natural fit between people who love to go to the gym and people whose bodies are set up to get the most benefit.

Yet everyone should move at least once an hour per day. If you sit still for an hour, blood fat and blood sugar levels mount. Just by getting out of your chair, standing up, and moving a bit, you help restore these levels to balance. If you add some walking, even moving at a slow pace will almost double your metabolism. Add a few minutes of vigorous exercise, enough to make your muscles warm, and you do even more to balance blood sugars. In other words, medical science supports the fact that our increasingly sedentary lifestyle isn't in harmony with how the body is designed to operate.

Yoga, which has become popular in the West, is a much broader regimen than physical conditioning (properly called hatha yoga). Its overall aim is to unite body, mind, and spirit into a harmonious whole. You can begin anywhere, because the whole system is interconnected. Settling the mind also settles the body, and vice versa. As long as you pay attention to the theme of "balance," you are benefiting every cell, allowing it to swing back and forth between rest and activity, pressure and release, high function and low function. The one thing that throws balance off the most is stasis. It may seem as if you are doing nothing when you sit around, but neglect isn't nothing. You are forcing your body to maintain low function all day, when what it wants is a dynamic balance of activity and rest.

As a program for balance, yoga can encompass any activity that helps bring a sense of peace and unity into your life. You deserve to relish the experience of being in a body. There are many ways to deepen the experience. Dancing, swimming, running, walking in the park—if they bring enjoyment, these activities can be like moving meditations for your body. Allow yourself to experience the richness of the natural world, strengthening your cardiovascular system, releasing endorphins in the brain, and clearing your mind. The ultimate purpose of yoga, in all its forms, is to enliven awareness and expand your understanding of the true self. So change all your preconceptions about exercise as a duty. Exercise is whatever body movement makes you feel more in touch with yourself and happier to be in the world.

Here's the centering thought for today's meditation: *I am flexible, strong, and balanced.*

Begin your meditation, following the instructions from Day 1.

The mantra: Now, gently introduce today's mantra: *Om Varunam Namah,* which means "My life is in harmony with cosmic law."

Follow through: As you continue with your day, contemplate this centering thought: *When I move, I enjoy being physical and the well-being this brings. When I move, I enjoy being physical and the well-being this brings.*

Saturday, Day 7
Your Well-Being

Congratulations! You've spent six days shifting your awareness to a more holistic view, not just intellectually but in practice. The goal of the Indian spiritual tradition is compatible with a holistic lifestyle. The word *yoga* means "unity," and yet the concept behind the word—being at one—is universal. Despite the differences in language and culture, every generation has contemplated how to reach fulfillment. The solutions they found were meant to be shared as a common inheritance. It would be a triumph of the human spirit if we ignored walls and boundaries, looking at *Aham Brahmasmi,* "I am the universe," as a vision applicable to everyone, not just the Vedic culture that flourished thousands of years ago. In the same way, Jesus' teaching about seeking the kingdom of heaven within is a solution that doesn't deserve to be sealed into a compartment only accessible to Christians.

You are seeking to find your own state of well-being, and yet in countless ways you are not alone. Every man and woman who has preceded you gave you a silent gift: the evolution of the brain. It has taken tens of thousands of years to create the mind-body connection as it exists today, balancing the primal impulses we share with reptiles, the emotions that began to appear among primates and early hominids, and the rationality and insight of the neocortex, the latest stage of the evolving brain.

In modern terms these daily meditations have been a new way to train the brain, but in the end, mind and spirit count the most. The brain is their physical interface, bringing purpose and meaning into the physical world so that each of us can write our own story. Meditation isn't an end unto itself. It brings your awareness to a place where you can make choices that determine how your story turns out, day by day. If you want lightness, balance, energy, and purity to be part of your story, writing them in begins now—they belong to the present moment.

You have all the tools you need to find your own fulfillment. What these daily meditations have added is a boost of inspiration. Today, we add the final grace note, which is gratitude. Gratitude is an important part of living in perfect balance. When we're grateful for everything we have in our lives, the ego steps out of the way, and we're completely open to the dynamic exchange of the universe. If you're not doing so already, begin keeping a gratitude journal and take note of everything you're grateful for each day. Take stock of how "awareness living" manifests in your life. Ask yourself how making conscious choices has created a difference. Thank yourself for all the changes you've made—large and small—and appreciate how they benefit you.

Remember, too, that we thrive in communion with others. So, share your new self-awareness, reach out to help others on their journey, and ask for support on yours. You are part of the collective consciousness, a wave in a vast and beautiful ocean. Acknowledge and celebrate your sacred connections.

Here's the centering thought for today's meditation: *I write my life story. I create my well-being.*

Begin your meditation, following the instructions from Day 1.

The mantra: Now, gently introduce today's mantra. It is *Sat, Chit, Ananda,* or "Being, consciousness, bliss."

Follow through: As you continue with your day, contemplate this centering thought: *My story is being perfected at this moment. My story is being perfected at this moment.*

PART THREE

RECIPES FROM THE CHOPRA CENTER KITCHEN

Recipes for Purity, Energy, and Balance

For this section I've asked the cooks at the Chopra Center to provide some of their favorite recipes to illustrate the kind of eating outlined in the chapter "What Should I Eat?" Each recipe has been tested thoroughly and been enjoyed by the wide range of people who come to the center. One of the highlights of their stay, they tell us, is the delicious food.

The recipes follow Ayurvedic principles. Some include all six tastes, although really it's the meal that needs to include them, not every single dish. The more important thing is to eat pure, wholesome food that leaves you feeling energetic and your body working in a state of balance. Those three themes—purity, energy, and balance—can be achieved through all kinds of menus; we're just giving you a head start here.

I realize that modern people lead busy lives, so I asked the cooks to give options for using canned or frozen ingredients when there isn't time to shop for fresh. Eating is for pleasure, not for putting stress on you, the cook, or inducing panic if everything isn't exactly perfect. Be easy with yourself. Changing your diet is a marathon, not a sprint. Don't get into the bad habit of blaming yourself for slipping up or backsliding—in fact, rid your vocabulary of these words. The stress you create by judging yourself negatively is far worse on your body than a guilty pleasure here and there.

If you're pressed for time, try to resist the option of fast food, though. These recipes allow you to change the trend in your diet, so that you develop your own repertoire of simple, wholesome dishes, even using a frozen vegetable or two. Another note from our cooks: When buying soy products, such as tofu or soymilk, as well as corn and corn-based products, always make sure that they haven't been genetically modified. Look for the seal from the Non-GMO Project, a nonprofit organization that offers third-party verification and labeling.

In my own life, which is filled with travel to destinations where the local eating scene is unknown, I have learned to enjoy the challenge of finding the freshest food, and usually the simplest. I have one full meal a day. A bowl of soup is enough in the evening. But it's a highlight when I'm able to settle in and eat at the Chopra Center. I come away inspired by how good it feels to combine taste, nature's abundance, and the kind of well-being that promises to sustain mind and body for a lifetime.

Light Breakfast

Morning Bliss Shake

Serves 1

5 whole almonds, skin on, soaked overnight in ½ cup water
2 teaspoons organic raw honey or maple syrup
1 ounce soy protein powder, plain or vanilla
Pinch of ground cinnamon
1 cup vanilla soymilk
1 medium banana, peeled and sliced
1 tablespoon aloe vera juice

Drain the almonds and discard the water. Place almonds in a blender, add the other ingredients, and blend until smooth. Take as a morning protein supplement and digestive aid.

Tofu Scramble

Prepared with fresh vegetables, fragrant herbs, and tofu, this recipe is delicious and satisfying at any time of day. To make a breakfast burrito to go, add a little cheese and salsa to the tofu mixture and wrap inside a warm whole-grain tortilla.

Serves 4

16 ounces fresh tofu, firm or extra firm, drained and crumbled
1 teaspoon olive oil
½ cup chopped leeks or onions
1 tablespoon Bragg Liquid Aminos or tamari
Pinch of black pepper
1 teaspoon ground cumin
1 teaspoon curry powder
½ teaspoon ground coriander
½ teaspoon dill
¼ teaspoon nutmeg
½ cup diced tomatoes
½ cup diced zucchini
1 cup fresh spinach
Vegetable stock
¼ cup chopped fresh cilantro

Place the crumbled tofu into a bowl and set aside. Heat a large sauté pan over medium heat and add the olive oil, leeks, liquid aminos, pepper, cumin, curry powder, coriander, dill, and nutmeg. Sauté for 2 minutes.

Add the tomatoes, zucchini, and spinach and continue to sauté until the vegetables begin to soften, about 5 minutes. Add some vegetable stock if the mixture becomes dry. Add the crumbled tofu and stir until well combined. Continue to sauté until the tofu is heated through. Garnish with the chopped cilantro.

Appetizers

Garden Spring Rolls

Makes 8 to 10 rolls

1 head butter lettuce
1 cup grated carrot
1 cup grated jicama*
1 cup cucumber, thinly sliced and chopped
1 cup zucchini, thinly sliced and chopped
½ cup radish or sunflower sprouts
¼ cup chopped fresh cilantro
¼ cup chopped fresh mint
¼ cup chopped fresh basil
1 cup shredded red cabbage (optional)

*Note: If jicama isn't available in your area, you can substitute crunchy Asian pears, crisp apples, water chestnuts, white turnips, or radishes.

Separate 8 to 10 of the largest lettuce leaves. Shred or thinly slice the rest of the lettuce. Combine the shredded lettuce with the carrot, jicama, cucumber, zucchini, and sprouts in a bowl. Add the fresh herbs and toss with ½ cup dressing (see the recipe that follows).

Bring a few cups of water to a boil in a saucepan. Quickly wilt the lettuce leaves by dipping them into the water for 10 to 15 seconds. Place the leaves in ice water for a minute, then remove and pat dry. Lay out the leaves on a paper towel on a flat surface. Divide the vegetables between all of the leaves. Roll them into small rolls, about 1 inch wide and 3 inches long. Display on a bed of shredded red cabbage (if using) and serve with dipping sauce and extra dressing (see the recipes that follow).

Dressing

½ cup apple juice
½ cup rice vinegar
¼ cup maple syrup or honey
1 teaspoon sesame seeds
½ teaspoon powdered or minced fresh ginger
1 tablespoon Bragg Liquid Aminos or tamari

Combine the ingredients and stir.

Spicy Lime and Red Pepper Dipping Sauce

Serves 4

¼ cup roasted red bell pepper, diced
¼ cup fresh lime juice (orange juice also works well)
2 tablespoons rice vinegar
2 tablespoons maple syrup
1 tablespoon Bragg Liquid Aminos or tamari
½ teaspoon cayenne pepper
1 tablespoon thinly chopped fresh basil
1 tablespoon peanut butter

Purée the ingredients in a blender until smooth. You may add a little orange juice or apple juice if you want to dilute the mixture.

Soups

Tomato Basil Soup

Serves 4 to 6

½ cup garbanzos, sorted, rinsed and soaked overnight in water, or
 one 14-ounce can, rinsed and drained
2 bay leaves
1 teaspoon olive oil
1 cup chopped leeks, shallots, or onions
1 tablespoon Italian herb mix
½ teaspoon black pepper
1 teaspoon fresh dill
1 tablespoon Bragg Liquid Aminos or tamari
1 cup cubed red bell pepper
1 cup zucchini, halved lengthwise and sliced
1 large tomato, chopped
2 cups tomato juice
2 cups vegetable stock
½ cup fresh basil leaves, packed

Drain and rinse the garbanzos and place in a soup pot. Add enough water to cover the beans by 2 inches. Bring to a boil, add the bay leaves, and then reduce the heat to a low rolling boil. Cook the beans until they are tender, 40 to 50 minutes. Drain the beans and set aside.

Heat the olive oil in a soup pot. Add the leeks, herb mix, black pepper, dill, and liquid aminos. Sauté for 3 to 4 minutes. Add the bell pepper and the zucchini. Sauté for another 5 minutes. Add the tomato and continue to sauté for another 3 to 4 minutes. Add the garbanzos and simmer for another 5 minutes, stirring frequently. Add the tomato juice and the vegetable stock. Bring to a boil. Reduce the heat. Slice the basil leaves thinly, add to the soup, and simmer for another 4 to 5 minutes. Remove the bay leaves before serving.

Vegetable Barley Soup

Although barley soup is traditionally made with beef, in this delicious recipe, vegetables and lentils create a rich flavor and texture without the additional fat. This is also a low-sugar recipe that is suitable for those with diabetes. Don't let the long list of ingredients intimidate you—most of the ingredients are spices that blend to create a fragrant, tasty soup.

Serves 4

1 teaspoon olive oil
1 teaspoon brown or yellow mustard seeds
Pinch of crushed red pepper flakes or chili powder
½ teaspoon black pepper
1 cup chopped leeks or onions
1 cup celery, sliced into ¼-inch pieces

1 tablespoon Bragg Liquid Aminos or tamari
1 cup lentils
½ cup pearl barley, rinsed and drained
1 teaspoon ground cumin
1 teaspoon ground coriander
½ teaspoon ground allspice
1 cup diced carrot
1 cup red or russet potato, cut into small cubes
1 teaspoon dried marjoram
4 to 6 cups vegetable stock
2 bay leaves
3 cups coarsely torn spinach or arugula or both
¼ cup chopped fresh parsley

Heat the olive oil in a soup pot over medium-high heat. Add the mustard seeds and allow them to pop briefly in the hot oil. Add the red pepper flakes, black pepper, leeks, celery, and liquid aminos. Then add the lentils.

Sauté until the leeks are translucent, 2 to 3 minutes. Add the barley and stir until well combined. Add the cumin, coriander, and allspice and continue to sauté for another 2 to 3 minutes, or until the barley browns slightly. Stir frequently. Add the carrot, potato, and marjoram. Simmer for another 3 minutes. Add some vegetable stock if the mixture gets dry.

When well browned, add 4 cups vegetable stock and the bay leaves. Bring to a boil, then reduce the heat and simmer until the carrot and potato are cooked and the barley is soft. Add the spinach. Add more vegetable stock if necessary as the barley absorbs the liquid. Remove the bay leaves before serving.

Garnish with fresh chopped parsley.

Mexican Tortilla Soup
with Avocado and Cilantro

Made with heating spices, fresh vegetables, crunchy tortilla strips, and a full-bodied broth, the Chopra Center's rendition of this classic recipe will warm you from the inside out.

Serves 4

2 teaspoons olive oil
1 cup chopped leeks or red onion
1 teaspoon Bragg Liquid Aminos or tamari
1 teaspoon black pepper
½ teaspoon crushed red pepper flakes
1 teaspoon mild chili powder
1 teaspoon ground cumin
1 teaspoon ground coriander
1 teaspoon dried marjoram
1 cup diced carrot
½ cup chopped green bell pepper
4 cups vegetable stock
1 cup corn, fresh or frozen (use organic if possible)
¼ cup roasted red bell pepper, chopped
2 corn tortillas, cut into 1-inch strips
¼ cup chopped fresh cilantro
1 cup cubed fresh avocado
Several cilantro sprigs with stems (for garnish)

In a soup pot, heat 1 teaspoon of the olive oil and add the leeks. Add the liquid aminos, black pepper, red pepper flakes, chili powder, cumin, coriander, and marjoram. Sauté for 1 minute. Next, add the carrot and bell pepper. Sauté for 2 minutes and then add ½ cup of the vegetable stock. Continue to simmer for 4 to 5 minutes. Add the corn, roasted bell pepper, and the rest of the vegetable stock. Allow the soup to simmer until the carrot is almost soft.

In a small sauté pan, heat the remaining 1 teaspoon olive oil and add the tortilla strips. Quickly stir-fry the tortilla strips until they become crisp. Remove from the heat and stir the tortilla strips into the soup along with the cilantro. Divide the avocado among individual bowls. Ladle the soup over the avocado and garnish with the cilantro sprigs. Serve right away.

Mulligatawny Soup

Serves 4

1 tablespoon olive oil
1 teaspoon brown or yellow mustard seeds
1½ cups chopped leeks or onions
1 cup chopped celery
4½ cups vegetable stock
1 tablespoon Bragg Liquid Aminos or tamari
½ teaspoon cayenne pepper or crushed red pepper flakes
1 large carrot, chopped
1 large potato, cubed
1 medium red bell pepper, chopped
1 medium green bell pepper, chopped
1 large tomato, chopped
1 teaspoon turmeric
1 teaspoon ground coriander
1 tablespoon ground cumin
½ teaspoon salt

1 teaspoon black pepper
1 cup coconut milk
2 to 4 tablespoons lemon juice
¼ bunch chopped fresh cilantro leaves
½ cup toasted shredded coconut (fresh if possible)

Heat the olive oil in a large soup pot. Pop the mustard seeds in the heated oil, then add the following ingredients in order, allowing 2 minutes between each to sauté: leeks, celery, ½ cup of the vegetable stock, liquid aminos, and cayenne pepper. Add the carrot, potato, bell peppers, tomato, turmeric, coriander, cumin, salt, black pepper, and the remaining 4 cups vegetable stock and sauté briefly. Simmer for 20 minutes. Add the coconut milk and lemon juice before serving. Garnish the bowls of soup with the cilantro and coconut.

Sweet Potato Ginger Soup

This recipe takes advantage of the sweet potato's naturally sweet flavor and enhances it with the refreshing taste of ginger and other herbs. Sweet potatoes are extremely nutritious, with high levels of iron, calcium, complex carbohydrates, and vitamins A, C, and B$_6$.

Serves 4

1 teaspoon olive oil
Pinch of crushed red pepper flakes
1 cup chopped leeks or onions
1 tablespoon minced fresh ginger or 1 teaspoon powdered ginger
2 tablespoons Bragg Liquid Aminos or tamari
5 cups sweet potatoes, peeled and cubed

1 teaspoon ground coriander
1 teaspoon garam masala
6 cups vegetable stock
¼ cup chopped fresh cilantro

Heat the olive oil in a soup pot over medium-high heat. Add the red pepper flakes, leeks, ginger, and liquid aminos. Sauté for 2 to 3 minutes. Add the sweet potatoes and sauté until they are well coated and begin to brown slightly. Add the coriander and garam masala. Sauté another 2 minutes, stirring frequently. Add the vegetable stock to cover the sweet potatoes and bring to a boil. Reduce the heat and simmer until the sweet potatoes are tender to the fork, testing after 5 minutes. Blend with a hand blender or food processor until the mixture has a smooth consistency, adding more stock as necessary. Reheat before serving and garnish with the cilantro.

Thai Squash Soup

Serves 4 to 6

1 large spaghetti squash, seeded and cleaned (any winter squash will
    work well)
1 teaspoon olive oil
2 cups chopped leeks
½ teaspoon crushed red pepper flakes
1 tablespoon minced fresh ginger
1 teaspoon Bragg Liquid Aminos or tamari
½ cup apple juice
2 medium stalks of lemongrass, cut into 4-inch lengths
2 teaspoons ground coriander

1 teaspoon ground cumin
4 to 5 cups vegetable stock (enough to cover the vegetables)
1 12-ounce can coconut milk
¼ cup thinly sliced fresh mint
¼ cup thinly sliced fresh basil

Preheat the oven to 350°F.

Cut the squash in half, remove the seeds, and lay the squash cut side down in a baking pan. Add about an inch of water and cover with foil. Bake for about 1 hour, or until soft. When the squash is cool enough to handle, remove the skin and cut the squash into 2-inch pieces. (You can also roast the squash: Peel it and chop it into 2-inch pieces and toss with 1 tablespoon sesame oil, 1 teaspoon ground cumin, and 1 teaspoon coriander. Lay the pieces on a baking sheet and then bake for 30 minutes. Let cool.)

In a soup pot, heat the olive oil. Add the leeks, red pepper flakes, and ginger and sauté.

Add the liquid aminos and baked squash pieces and bring to a simmer. Add the apple juice, lemongrass, coriander, and cumin. Simmer for 3 minutes. Add enough vegetable stock to just cover the squash and simmer for 10 to 15 minutes. Remove the lemongrass. Use a hand blender or food processor to purée the soup until smooth, adding some of the coconut milk to each batch. Divide the soup into individual bowls and garnish with the mint and basil.

Very Simple Pumpkin Soup

Serves 4 to 6

Pumpkins are a winter squash with a sweet flavor. The cheerful pumpkin's orange flesh is also packed with beta-carotene, an antioxidant that helps improve immune function and reduce the risk of cancer and heart disease. A cup of cooked pumpkin has just 49 calories, 2.7 grams of fiber, 567 milligrams of potassium, and 5,116 micrograms of vitamin A.

1 large pumpkin (about 3 pounds), or 3 cups canned pumpkin
1 teaspoon olive oil
1 cup chopped leeks or onions
½ teaspoon black pepper
1 teaspoon ground cinnamon
1 teaspoon ground cumin
1 teaspoon curry powder
½ teaspoon ground cloves
2 to 3 cups vegetable stock
1 tablespoon Bragg Liquid Aminos or tamari
1 cup soymilk
½ teaspoon vanilla extract (optional)
Ground nutmeg

If using fresh pumpkin, preheat the oven to 350°F. Wash the pumpkin, cut it in half, and remove the seeds (reserve them for roasting; See "Tip," page 259). Place the pumpkin halves cut side down in a baking pan. Pour in 1½ cups water and cover the pan with foil. Bake for 30 minutes, or until a knife inserted in the pumpkin pulls out easily. Let cool, then remove the pumpkin pulp from the rind with a spoon. Place the pulp into a bowl and set aside. You should have about 3 cups of pumpkin pulp.

Heat a soup pot over medium heat and add the olive oil. Add the leeks, pepper, cinnamon, cumin, curry powder, and cloves. Sauté until the leeks are translucent, 4 to 5 minutes. Add some vegetable stock if the mixture begins to dry.

Add the pumpkin and continue to sauté for another 3 to 4 minutes. Add the liquid aminos and brown the pumpkin slightly. Add vegetable stock to cover the pumpkin and bring to a boil. Reduce the heat to low and simmer for about 10 minutes. Use a hand blender or food processor to purée the soup until smooth and creamy, adding some of the soymilk and vanilla (if using) to each batch. Return the soup to the pot and reheat if necessary. Garnish with a sprinkle of nutmeg.

Tip: Don't throw away the pumpkin seeds! You can make a tasty snack by roasting these hearty seeds, which are a good source of protein, zinc, and other vitamins. Place on a baking sheet and roast at 325°F until pale brown, tossing occasionally to ensure even browning. Watch carefully since nuts and seeds burn easily.

Spinach and Lentil Soup

Serves 4

1 teaspoon olive oil
1 cup chopped leeks or onions
1 cup celery, cut into ¼-inch slices
2 garlic cloves, minced, or ½ teaspoon garlic powder
1 teaspoon minced fresh ginger
Pinch of crushed red pepper flakes
½ teaspoon black pepper
1 teaspoon chopped fresh rosemary
1 tablespoon Bragg Liquid Aminos or tamari

1 cup diced carrot
½ cup bulgur (optional)
1 teaspoon ground cumin
½ teaspoon ground allspice
1 cup brown lentils, sorted, rinsed, and drained
5 to 6 cups vegetable stock
2 bay leaves
2 tablespoons tomato paste
4 cups coarsely chopped fresh spinach
¼ cup chopped fresh parsley
1 cup diced tomatoes

Heat a soup pot, add the olive oil, then add the leeks, celery, garlic, ginger, red pepper flakes, black pepper, and rosemary. Add the liquid aminos and carrot. Sauté for 3 minutes, then add the bulgur (if using) and sauté until golden brown. Add the cumin and allspice, stirring frequently. Add the lentils, 5 cups of the vegetable stock, and the bay leaves. Bring the soup to a boil, then reduce the heat and continue to simmer until the lentils are tender, 30 to 40 minutes. Add more vegetable stock as necessary. Add the tomato paste and spinach and simmer until the spinach is wilted, about 5 minutes. Remove the bay leaves before serving. Ladle into soup bowls and garnish with the fresh parsley and diced tomatoes.

Entrées and Side Dishes

Sautéed Greens and Cabbage

Serves 4 to 6

2 tablespoons olive oil
1 teaspoon minced fresh ginger
½ teaspoon turmeric
2 bunches Swiss chard or kale
1 small head cabbage
1 tablespoon ground coriander
1½ teaspoons salt
½ teaspoon black pepper

Heat the olive oil in a wok and sauté the ginger and turmeric for about 40 seconds. Add the Swiss chard and cabbage and toss over high heat for about 4 minutes. Sprinkle with the coriander, salt, and pepper and stir to coat the vegetables. Add ⅛ cup water, cover with a tight-fitting lid, and simmer for 5 to 7 minutes or until done to taste.

262 What Are You Hungry For?

Kicharee

Kicharee is a wonderfully balancing meal that is light, nourishing, and easy to digest.

Serves 4 to 6

⅓ cup split mung dal (mung beans)
⅔ cup basmati rice or other grain, such as quinoa or barley
½ teaspoon ground turmeric
1 tablespoon minced fresh ginger or ½ teaspoon ground ginger
½ teaspoon roasted cumin seeds
½ teaspoon ground coriander
1 to 2 cups seasonal vegetables, such as kale, Swiss chard, spinach,
    peas, seaweed, or mushrooms
1 teaspoon olive or hempseed oil

Place the mung dal, rice, and 3 to 4 cups water in a medium stockpot. Bring to a boil, then reduce the heat to low. Add the turmeric, cumin, ginger, and coriander and simmer, covered, over very low heat, stirring often so the mung beans do not scorch. The total timing will depend on the age and dryness of your beans; begin testing for softness after 15 to 20 minutes. Add extra water if necessary to keep the beans and rice moist. When the dal and rice are tender, add the seasonal vegetables and the oil to taste.

Curried Vegetables

Serves 2 to 4

3 tablespoons virgin coconut oil or olive oil
1 teaspoon cumin seeds
1 teaspoon coriander seeds
1 teaspoon fennel seeds
1 teaspoon brown or yellow mustard seeds
1 tablespoon chopped fresh ginger
Pinch of ground asafetida
2 to 3 cups chopped fresh vegetables of your choice
Ground cumin, turmeric, and cinnamon to taste
Coconut milk or yogurt (optional)

Heat the coconut oil in a large pan over medium-high heat. Add the cumin, coriander, fennel, and mustard seeds and sauté until the seeds are faintly brown and release a delicious aroma, around 1 minute. Add the ginger, asafetida, and chopped vegetables and sauté for a few seconds until the vegetables are coated in the spiced oil. Add ½ cup water or vegetable stock and simmer over low heat until done, about 15 minutes. Add ground cumin, turmeric, and cinnamon to taste. Add any "quick-to-cook" vegetables such as spinach and peas at the end and cook for 3 minutes. You can also add coconut milk or yogurt (if using) to make a creamier sauce.

Ratatouille Stew

Serves 4

1 large eggplant, peeled and diced
1 teaspoon olive oil
2 large leeks or onions, chopped
2 teaspoons Italian seasoning
1 teaspoon dried marjoram
1 teaspoon dried thyme
½ teaspoon black pepper
1 teaspoon garlic powder
1 tablespoon Bragg Liquid Aminos or tamari
2 large zucchini, cubed
3 large green and red bell peppers, cubed
2 cups diced tomatoes
1½ cups vegetable stock
½ cup thinly sliced fresh basil

Submerge the eggplant cubes in a bowl of water with a sprinkle of salt in it. Set aside. Heat the olive oil in a large soup pot over medium heat. Add the leeks, Italian seasoning, marjoram, thyme, black pepper, garlic powder, and liquid aminos and sauté briefly. Add the eggplant, zucchini, and bell peppers and sauté for 4 to 5 minutes. Add the tomatoes and continue to simmer another 3 to 4 minutes. Add the vegetable stock when the mixture begins to dry out. Simmer the stew over low heat for 20 to 30 minutes. Add the fresh basil just before serving.

Aloo Gobi

Aloo gobi is a spicy Indian dish traditionally made with cauliflower and potatoes. This delicious version includes a variety of nutrient-rich spices, such as turmeric, ginger, and cayenne pepper.

Serves 4 to 6

3 tablespoons olive oil
½ teaspoon minced fresh ginger
½ teaspoon turmeric
2 medium potatoes, peeled and cut into 1-inch cubes
1 medium cauliflower, cut into 1-inch florets
1 teaspoon ground cumin
1 teaspoon ground coriander
½ teaspoon cayenne pepper
1 teaspoon salt
4 tablespoons chopped fresh cilantro

Heat the olive oil in a large saucepan over medium heat. Add the ginger and turmeric and sauté for about 40 seconds. Add the potatoes, raise the heat to high, and sauté for 4 minutes. Then add the cauliflower, cumin, coriander, cayenne pepper, and salt and sauté for 8 minutes. Add 4 tablespoons water, cover with a tight-fitting lid, and steam till the vegetables are tender. Just before serving, add the cilantro.

Chili Chickpeas

Serves 4 to 8

2 cups cooked garbanzos, drained
1 tablespoon Thai-style chili paste
¼ teaspoon lemongrass
1 tablespoon Bragg Liquid Aminos or tamari
¼ cup light coconut milk
2 tablespoons finely chopped fresh cilantro

Heat a small sauté pan over medium heat. Add the garbanzos, chili paste, lemongrass, and liquid aminos. Cook, stirring frequently, until the chili paste is melted and the garbanzos begin to brown, about 10 minutes. Add the coconut milk and cook until somewhat thickened, about 5 minutes. Remove from the heat. Toss with the cilantro just before serving.

Quinoa Pilaf

Serves 4 to 6

Serve this dish alongside a main dish or as the star of the meal!

1 cup quinoa, cleaned and rinsed
2½ cups vegetable stock or water
1 teaspoon olive oil
Pinch of crushed red pepper flakes
½ teaspoon black pepper
1 cup chopped leeks or onions

1 teaspoon ground cumin

1 tablespoon Bragg Liquid Aminos or tamari

2 garlic cloves, minced (optional)

2 medium zucchini, halved lengthwise and sliced

1 medium yellow squash, halved lengthwise and sliced

2 handfuls mixed greens (Swiss chard, spinach, mustard greens),
  washed and torn into pieces

3 tablespoons chopped fresh cilantro

1 teaspoon fresh oregano

1 teaspoon chili powder or paprika

1 large tomato, diced

Toast the quinoa in a dry skillet, stirring frequently, until golden brown, about 2 minutes. Bring 2 cups of the vegetable stock to a boil. Add the quinoa and simmer until the liquid is absorbed, 15 to 20 minutes. Place the quinoa in a bowl and fluff with a fork. Set aside to cool.

In a sauté pan, heat the olive oil over medium heat; add the red pepper flakes, black pepper, leeks, cumin, liquid aminos, and garlic (if using). Sauté until the leeks are browned around the edges, about 5 minutes. Add the zucchini and yellow squash and sauté for 3 to 4 minutes, until the vegetables are just tender. Add the greens and continue to sauté until they are just wilted. Remove from the heat, draining any excess liquid, and set aside.

Add the cilantro, oregano, chili powder, and tomato to the quinoa. Stir together, then add the vegetable mixture. Toss together until well combined.

You can serve this recipe as a hot pilaf side dish or as a wonderful cold salad on a bed of greens.

Thai-Style Noodles (Pad Thai)

In Thailand, pad Thai has traditionally been a light noodle dish with a complex flavor created from a mixture of fresh spices. In its Western incarnation, pad Thai is often a heavy, oily dish with a strong emphasis on the sweet and salty tastes. This delicious recipe from the Chopra Center is based on the original, lighter version of the dish. Instead of stir-frying the noodles in a lot of oil, they are cooked with a little olive oil, vegetable stock, and a unique blend of spices and herbs.

Serves 4

16 ounces baked marinated tofu or tempeh (see the recipe on page 270) or 2 cups cooked, diced chicken (you can also substitute plain tofu if you prefer)

Thai Sauce
½ cup vegetable stock
¼ cup rice vinegar
2 tablespoons apple juice
2 teaspoons lemon juice
1 teaspoon miso paste
1 teaspoon paprika
1 teaspoon Chinese five-spice powder
1 tablespoon maple syrup
1 tablespoon Bragg Liquid Aminos or tamari
2 tablespoons thinly sliced fresh basil leaves

Noodles
8 ounces rice noodles or soba noodles
1 teaspoon olive or sesame oil

½ cup sliced leeks or onions

Pinch of crushed red pepper flakes

1 teaspoon ground coriander

2 tablespoons minced fresh ginger

1 garlic clove, minced (optional)

2 tablespoons vegetable stock

2 tablespoons toasted sliced almonds

¼ cup chopped green onions (scallions), white and green parts

2 cups mung bean sprouts, rinsed

½ cup chopped fresh cilantro

If you're using marinated tofu or tempeh, remove it from the marinade and cut it into 1-inch strips. Set aside.

In a blender, combine all of the Thai sauce ingredients and purée until smooth. Add the basil after blending. Set aside.

Cook or soak the noodles according to the package directions. Rinse, place in a large bowl, and sprinkle with additional oil to keep the noodles from sticking.

Tip: Soak the noodles only until they are slightly soft and pliable but not fully expanded. If you soak them until they are soft enough to eat, when you put them in the dish, they will turn to mush.

Heat the olive oil in a wok or large sauté pan. Add the leeks, red pepper flakes, coriander, ginger, and garlic (if using) and sauté for 2 minutes, adding the vegetable stock after 1 minute. Add the tofu, tempeh strips, or chicken. Cover, reduce the heat to low, and simmer for 3 to 4 minutes.

Add the almonds, green onions, bean sprouts, and cilantro. Simmer until heated through, 3 to 4 minutes. Add the sauce and simmer for another 2 to 3 minutes, then pour the mixture over the noodles and toss until well combined. Serve with steamed vegetables.

Simple Marinade for Tofu or Tempeh

Serves 4

1 16-ounce package fresh extra-firm tofu or tempeh
¾ cup Bragg Liquid Aminos or tamari
¾ cup rice vinegar
2 tablespoons balsamic vinegar
2 tablespoons maple syrup
1 teaspoon ground ginger
1 teaspoon ground cumin
½ teaspoon crushed red pepper flakes
1 teaspoon sesame oil

Slice the tofu or tempeh into ¼-inch slabs or cut into cubes. Combine the rest of the ingredients in a shallow baking pan. Add the tofu or tempeh. Soak overnight. To speed up the process, bake the tofu or tempeh at 350°F for 20 to 30 minutes, then cool. Remove the tofu or tempeh from the marinade and use in a variety of dishes. Store in a container with a tight-fitting lid.

The Very Best Tofu Burgers

Makes 8 burgers

2–3 slices dried bread
2 tablespoons olive oil
1 cup chopped leeks or onions
½ teaspoon black pepper
16 ounces fresh, low-fat tofu, firm or extra firm, drained and
   crumbled

¼ cup mixed nuts and seeds (sunflower seeds, walnuts, pine nuts,
    almonds, or others)
1 cup grated zucchini
1 cup grated carrot
1 teaspoon dried basil
1 teaspoon dried oregano
1 teaspoon dried thyme
1 teaspoon dried tarragon
1 teaspoon minced garlic or 1 teaspoon garlic powder
1 tablespoon Bragg Liquid Aminos or tamari

Preheat the oven to 350°F. Place the bread in a food processor and
pulse into bread crumbs, then set aside. Heat 1 tablespoon olive oil in
a small sauté pan over high heat. Add the leeks and pepper and sauté
for 2 to 3 minutes. Remove from the heat and cool. Place the tofu,
mixed nuts and seeds, zucchini, carrot, and sautéed leeks in a food
processor. Pulse a few times, then add the basil, oregano, thyme,
tarragon, garlic, and liquid aminos. Continue to pulse to a smooth
consistency. The mixture should be thick, yet firm.

Scoop out the mixture with a ½-cup measuring cup and form into
balls. Flatten the balls into burgers and coat each side with the bread
crumbs. Heat 1 tablespoon oil in a pan and sauté the patties briefly,
until golden brown, adding a bit more oil if it gets absorbed before
you brown the second side. Place on an oiled sheet pan and bake for
10 to 15 minutes, until firm. Serve on a bun or as an entrée with a
sauce of your choice.

Salads

Sour Citrus Berry Sunburst Salad

Serves 4

2 oranges, peeled and sectioned
1 cup sliced fresh strawberries
1 cup fresh raspberries or blackberries
1 cup fresh blueberries

Rinse and drain fruit well. Cut the orange slices in half. Prepare the dressing (see the recipe that follows) and place it in a large bowl. Place the oranges in the bowl and coat with the dressing. Remove from the bowl and arrange on a platter as the bottom layer. Reserve 10 pieces for garnish. Place the strawberries in the dressing and coat. Remove and arrange around the orange slices like the rays of a sun. Coat the raspberries, arrange on top of the oranges, and then coat the blueberries and arrange around the raspberries. You are creating a sunburst with the fruit. Drizzle the dressing on top of the fruit and garnish with the reserved orange pieces.

Dressing

¼ cup rice vinegar
¼ cup maple syrup or organic honey
1 tablespoon balsamic vinegar
1 teaspoon Bragg Liquid Aminos, tamari, or light soy sauce
½ teaspoon ground cinnamon
½ teaspoon ground ginger
½ cup apple juice

Combine all of the ingredients and mix well.

Goddess Greens with Gorgonzola

Serves 4 to 6

This delicious salad will nurture your love for sensory pleasures of the palate. The sweet, crunchy flavor of honey-glazed walnuts contrasts with the pungent Gorgonzola and fresh spinach. Enjoy as an appetizer or light entrée.

Serves 4 to 6

2 pounds fresh spinach, washed and stemmed
1 cup honey-glazed walnuts (see the recipe that follows)
½ cup crumbled Gorgonzola cheese
½ cup currants
3 tablespoons poppy seed dressing (see the recipe that follows)

Toss all of the ingredients together and arrange on chilled plates.

Honey-Glazed Walnuts

Makes 1 cup, or 4 to 6 servings

½ teaspoon olive oil
1 cup walnut pieces
1 tablespoon honey

Heat the olive oil in a skillet over medium heat (don't allow it to reach the smoking point). Toss in the walnuts and sauté until golden, about 2 minutes. Add the honey and coat the walnuts well. Let cool completely before using.

Poppy Seed Dressing

Makes about ¾ cup

1 tablespoon Dijon mustard
1 tablespoon olive oil
1 tablespoon honey
1 tablespoon Bragg Liquid Aminos or tamari
1 tablespoon lemon juice
½ cup orange juice
¼ cup plain yogurt
1 tablespoon poppy seeds

Combine all of the ingredients in a small jar and shake well. The dressing can be stored in the refrigerator for several days.

Chopra Center Tabouli

The vegetables, grains, and beans in this tasty salad provide a steady flow of energy that is particularly balancing for those who have a propensity to get irritable and overeat if they let themselves get too hungry.

Serves 4

1¾ cups vegetable stock or water
1 cup bulgur wheat
1 teaspoon olive oil
½ cup chopped leeks or onions
¼ cup roasted red bell pepper, chopped (fresh will also work well)
1 cup cubed zucchini
½ cup cooked dried or canned Great Northern beans (rinsed)
1 cup diced tomatoes
½ cup chopped fresh parsley or other fresh herb
2 tablespoons finely sliced fresh basil
½ cup chopped fresh mint
2 tablespoons kalamata olives, pitted and sliced

Bring 1½ cups of the vegetable stock to a boil in a small saucepan, then add the bulgur. Stir with a fork, remove from the heat, and cover with a tight-fitting lid. Allow the bulgur to soak for 15 minutes. Fluff with a fork, place in a large mixing bowl, and let cool.

Meanwhile, heat the olive oil in a sauté pan over medium heat. Add the leeks and sauté briefly. Add the bell pepper and zucchini and sauté for 2 more minutes. Add the beans and sauté for another 2 minutes. Add the remaining ¼ cup vegetable stock as the mixture begins to dry out. Remove from the heat and cool. Add the tomatoes, parsley, basil, mint, and olives to the cooled bulgur and mix.

Finally, pour the dressing (see the recipe that follows) over the bulgur mixture.

Dressing
2 tablespoons lemon juice
1 tablespoon apple juice
1 tablespoon Bragg Liquid Aminos or tamari
1 teaspoon dried dill
½ teaspoon salt
½ teaspoon black pepper
2 garlic cloves, minced, or ½ teaspoon garlic powder
2 teaspoons olive oil

In a small bowl, combine all of the ingredients except the olive oil. Whisk the mixture and then continue to stir as you slowly add the olive oil.

Variations
This recipe lends itself to infinite variety. You can substitute your own favorite chopped, grated, or shredded vegetables for those called for in this version of the recipe. For added flavor and texture, try adding currants, raisins, sunflower seeds, pine nuts, or feta cheese. Enjoy!

Kashi Salad

Serves 4 to 6

1 cup diced carrot
1 cup diced celery
½ cup roasted red bell pepper, diced
¾ cups mixed beans, cooked and cooled (can use any kind of beans
    and legumes: peas, lentils, adzuki beans, and so on)
4 cups cooked kashi
¼ cup toasted pine nuts
½ cup toasted sunflower seeds
⅛ cup red wine vinegar
1 tablespoon sesame oil
⅛ cup prepared mustard
⅛ cup Bragg Liquid Aminos or tamari
¼ teaspoon black pepper
1 tablespoon olive oil

In a large bowl, combine the carrot, celery, bell pepper, beans, kashi, pine nuts, and sunflower seeds. In another bowl, mix the vinegar, sesame oil, mustard, liquid aminos, black pepper, and olive oil and toss into the salad.

Condiments, Dips, and Sauces

Cucumber Raita

Serves 4

3 small cucumbers, peeled, seeded, and diced
2 tablespoons lemon juice
1 teaspoon ground cumin
½ teaspoon dried dill
Pinch of salt
2 teaspoons chopped fresh cilantro
1 cup plain low-fat yogurt

Place the cucumbers in a small bowl. Add the lemon juice, cumin, dill, salt, and cilantro and toss gently. Add the yogurt and combine with a fork. Serve as a condiment with curry or as a dressing for salads and wraps.

Sprouted Chickpea Hummus

Makes 3 cups

2 cups sprouted chickpeas
1 tablespoon sunflower oil
3 tablespoons lemon juice
½ teaspoon freshly ground black pepper
½ teaspoon ground paprika
½ cup grated carrot
½ cup finely chopped fresh parsley
Salt to taste

Put the chickpeas, sunflower oil, lemon juice, pepper, and paprika in a food processor fitted with a stainless-steel blade. Process until the mixture forms a fairly smooth paste. Transfer the mixture to a bowl, stir in the carrot and parsley, and season to taste with the salt.

Easy Curry Masala

Makes 1½ to 2 cups

This simple sauce can be used with many vegetable combinations. It can also be used for grilled tofu or as the base of a soup.

2 tablespoons olive oil
1 cup chopped leeks or white onions
1 tablespoon fresh ginger, minced, or 1 teaspoon ground ginger
1 teaspoon ground cumin
½ teaspoon cayenne pepper or crushed red pepper flakes
½ teaspoon turmeric
1 large ripe tomato, finely chopped
1 tablespoon Bragg Liquid Aminos or tamari

Heat the olive oil in a medium saucepan over medium heat. Add the leeks and ginger and sauté. Add the cumin, cayenne pepper, turmeric, and tomato and sauté for 1 minute. Add the liquid aminos and simmer for 2 minutes.

Pungent Mango Tomato Salsa

Makes 1½ to 2 cups

1 whole mild Anaheim chili, roasted and peeled, or use ¼ cup
    canned mild green chilies
1 ripe mango, cubed
2 medium ripe tomatoes, cubed
1 tablespoon Bragg Liquid Aminos, tamari, or soy sauce
1 medium onion or leek, chopped
2 garlic cloves, minced, or 1 teaspoon minced fresh ginger
1 tablespoon lemon juice
¼ cup chopped fresh cilantro
1 teaspoon ground cumin
½ teaspoon ground coriander

To roast a chili:

Using a pair of stainless-steel tongs, hold the raw chili over the di-rect flame of a gas burner. Allow the flame to char the skin of the chili until it blisters. Carefully turn the chili continuously to char as much surface area as possible. Place the charred chili in a paper bag. The chili will steam inside the paper bag, loosening the charred skin. Allow the chili to steam until cool enough to handle, about 10 minutes. Peel off the skin under running water.

To assemble the salsa:

Chop up the chili and place it in a bowl. Add the mango and tomatoes and set aside. Heat the liquid aminos in a medium saucepan over
low heat. Add the onion and garlic and sauté very briefly. Add the
onion mixture to the mango mixture. Add the lemon juice, cilantro,
cumin, and coriander and toss well. Chill for 1 hour before serving.
Add 1 teaspoon liquid aminos if a more salty taste is desired.

Mint Chutney

Makes 1 cup

1 cup plain yogurt, preferably low-fat
Bunch of fresh cilantro
2-inch piece ginger, peeled
1 serrano chili
1 teaspoon salt
1 teaspoon ground cumin
½ teaspoon granulated sugar
¼ cup fresh mint leaves (no stems)

Place all of the ingredients in a blender and blend until the chutney
has a fine consistency. Serve at room temperature.

Fresh Pesto and Almonds

Makes 1 cup

1 small leek
½ cup almonds
2 cups lightly packed fresh basil leaves
½ cup olive oil
½ cup lemon juice
1 teaspoon black pepper

Cut off and discard the green parts of the leek and trim off the base. Quarter the white part lengthwise and wash thoroughly under running water to remove any dirt and sand. Drain. Roughly chop the leek into chunks. Place the almonds in a food processor and pulse several times. Add the leek and remaining ingredients and blend until smooth.

Serving Suggestions
Toss with fresh pasta.
Use as a pizza topping.
Serve with plain rice.
Spread on sandwiches in place of mustard or mayonnaise.
Add to Italian soup for extra flavor.

Desserts

Berry Yogurt Parfait

Serves 4

1 pint fresh berries or 10 ounces frozen berries
½ teaspoon ground cloves
½ teaspoon ground cinnamon
2 cups plain yogurt, preferably low-fat
1 teaspoon vanilla extract
2 tablespoons maple syrup or organic honey

In a small sauté pan, warm the berries, adding a little water as needed to prevent burning. Simmer for 1 to 2 minutes. Add the cloves and cinnamon and continue to simmer until the berries begin to soften, 3 to 5 minutes. Remove from the heat and place in a mixing bowl to cool slightly. If the berries produce too much liquid, spoon them into the bowl with a slotted spoon.

Add the yogurt and vanilla and mix well. Sweeten to taste with maple syrup. Serve with granola or hot cereal for breakfast or enjoy as a light dessert or snack.

The Chopra Center's Unbelievable Double Chocolate Cake

Applesauce and tofu give this chocolate cake a rich, moist texture without the many grams of saturated fat contained in traditional recipes. It is an excellent dessert for celebrations with loved ones.

Serves 12

12 ounces low-fat silken tofu, firm or extra-firm, crumbled and
   drained for 20 minutes
¼ cup canola oil
1 cup maple syrup
¾ cup applesauce
2 teaspoons vanilla extract
1 cup whole-wheat pastry flour
¾ cup unsweetened cocoa powder
2 teaspoons baking powder
1 teaspoon baking soda
1 cup chocolate chips

Preheat the oven to 350°F.

Oil an 8-inch round pan or a 9-by-13-inch pan and set aside. Use a food processor or blender to purée the tofu, canola oil, maple syrup, applesauce, and vanilla until smooth. Set aside.

In a large bowl, sift together the flour, cocoa powder, baking powder, and baking soda. Pour the wet ingredients into the dry ingredients and combine. Gently fold in the chocolate chips, being careful not to overmix.

Pour the batter into the prepared baking pan and bake for 30 to 40 minutes, or until an inserted toothpick comes out clean. Once the cake cools, ice it (see the recipe that follows).

Chocolate Icing
1 cup unsalted butter
4 cups chocolate chips
1 12-ounce package silken tofu
¼ cup maple syrup

Melt the butter and chocolate chips in a saucepan over low heat and stir until smooth. In a food processor or mixer, blend the tofu and maple syrup. Add the melted butter and chocolate to the tofu mixture. Allow the icing to cool to room temperature before frosting the cake.

Vegan Oatmeal Cookies

These flavorful cookies have a wonderful soft, chewy texture created by the mixture of mango, coconut, oats, and dried fruit.

Makes 20 to 22 cookies

½ cup mango purée
1 cup turbinado sugar
2 tablespoons maple syrup
1 teaspoon vanilla extract
1 cup rolled oats
1 cup unbleached or spelt flour
1 cup dates or other dried fruit
1 cup raisins
1 cup coconut flakes
½ teaspoon baking soda
1 teaspoon ground cinnamon
1 teaspoon ground allspice

Preheat the oven to 350°F.

Grease baking sheets or spray them with vegetable oil. Combine the mango purée, sugar, maple syrup, and vanilla. In a separate large bowl, combine all of the other ingredients. Mix the wet ingredients into the dry ingredients with your bare hands.

Use a ¼-cup measure to portion out the dough and roll it into balls. Place on the prepared baking sheets and bake for 15 minutes, until golden brown.

Beverages

Ginger Tea

Ginger tea is a powerful cleansing drink that removes toxins and restores balance to the body. It also benefits the digestive system and helps diminish cravings for sweet and salty foods. The Chopra Center recommends drinking two to three cups of hot ginger tea every day.

To make 1 quart of ginger tea:
Chop an unpeeled 2-inch piece of whole ginger into coarse pieces and place in a 2- to 3-quart pot with 1 quart purified water. Bring to a boil, then reduce the heat and allow the tea to simmer for 15 minutes. Strain the tea and store in a thermos bottle or glass jar.

To make 1 cup of ginger tea:
Take a piece of whole, unpeeled ginger root and grate 1 heaping teaspoon. Stir the ginger into a cup of hot water and let steep for 2 minutes. Strain or let the ginger settle at the bottom of the cup.

Sweet Lassi

Lassi is traditionally served at the end of a meal to aid digestion. It is
best consumed in warmer weather.

Serves 4 to 6

1 cup plain yogurt, preferably low-fat
¼ cup granulated sugar or honey
2 to 3 cups cold filtered water
¼ teaspoon ground cardamom
2 teaspoons rose water (optional)

Combine all of the ingredients in a large jar and shake, or place in a
blender and blend for about 30 seconds.

Refrigerate for 30 minutes before serving.

Acknowledgments

A new book makes me feel how fortunate I am to see my words reach publication as if by the touch of a button. There is no button, of course, but the dedicated work of many people behind the scenes. Thanking them here is a small token of the appreciation they deserve.

The team at Harmony Crown has stood by me and believed in my work even as the publishing industry goes through anxious changes. Tina Constable, publisher at Crown, Mauro DiPreta, Tara Gilbride, Meredith McGinnis, and Ayelet Gruenspecht have been unswerving supporters.

Gary Jansen, aided by Amanda O'Connor, has proven many times over what it means for a writer to be backed by a talented, enthusiastic editor. Our relationship has become one of trust, affection, and mutual respect.

The seed for this book was planted by Bob Marty, who went on to develop it as a program on PBS. Many thanks for your creativity and enthusiasm.

My day-to-day life is expertly managed by the inspiring Chopra Center staff, who are as near and dear as family, beginning with Carolyn and Felicia Rangel. For the special needs of this book, I must also thank Sara Harvey, Kathy Bankerd, Kyla Stinnett, Teresa

Long, and Attila Ambrus. You have all taught me what "the spirit in action" means.

Since we came to the United States in 1970 as newlyweds, my wife, Rita, and I have had the joy of seeing our family grow. Now it embraces Mallika, Sumant, Tara, Leela, Gotham, Candice, and Krishu.

Let these brief thanks stand in for how much I owe you and how deeply you are appreciated.